THE TOPIC OF CANCER

THE
TOPIC
OF
CANCER

IRA PILGRIM

THOMAS Y. CROWELL COMPANY
ESTABLISHED 1834   NEW YORK

ACKNOWLEDGMENTS

I wish to thank the following sources for permission to use material in this book:

The Connecticut Tumor Registry of the Connecticut State Department of Health for tables from "Cancer in Connecticut Mortality Data."

St. Martin's Press, Inc., Macmillan & Co., Ltd., for quotation from *Calculus Made Easy* by Silvanus P. Thompson.

The Viking Press for part of a poem by James Weldon Johnson from *God's Trombones*.

The quotes from the book of Job are from *The Jerusalem Bible*, Doubleday & Company. Inc., Garden City, N.Y.. 1966.

DESIGNED BY ABIGAIL MOSELEY
MANUFACTURED IN THE UNITED STATES OF AMERICA

1 2 3 4 5 6 7 8 9 10

LIBRARY OF CONGRESS CATALOGING IN PUBLICATION DATA

Pilgrim, Ira.
    The topic of cancer.

    Includes bibliographical references.
    1. Cancer.   I. Title.   [DNLM: 1. Neoplasms—Popular works. QZ201 P638t 1974]
RC263.P56 1974   616.9'94   74-7500
ISBN 0-690-00516-4

I am deeply grateful to the American public, who paid for my education, research, and the time to write this book.*

* I was going to dedicate this book to the National Cancer Institute; but then I remembered a time when I applied for a government contract. In the contract proposal, I stated that "the laboratory would be operated as a public service." The people who reviewed the application hit the ceiling; and the remark that came back to me was, "What does he mean—a public service—he's doing this for the government."

Preface

When someone asks me what I do for a living, and I reply that I am doing cancer research, the next question is invariably, "Are they going to find a cure?" My usual reply is to rephrase the question and say, "If you mean will cancer go the way of smallpox or pneumonia in the foreseeable future—the answer is that it probably will not."

I have never been satisfied with that oversimplified answer, but it is hard—if not impossible—to explain the problems involved in studying the cause and treatment of cancer while standing with a cocktail glass in your hand.

The image that most people have of the cancer scientist is that he is a physician who is frantically battling to find "the answer" to "the disease" that is killing his patient. We often picture the scientists as working at a frantic pace, surrounded by a continual life-and-death drama; in short he is the image of Paul Muni as Dr. Louis Pasteur, Dr. Martin Arrowsmith, Dr. James Kildare, and Dr. Ben Casey all rolled into one. We read articles in the newspapers which lead us to imagine someone in a white coat, with a test tube in his hand, holding it up to the window and saying, "Here, gentlemen, is the cancer virus!"

In fact, it is not this way at all. The things that scientists get excited about are not in the same league as the prevention of smallpox by vaccination with material from a cow, nor the transplantation of a heart. The exciting developments in cancer research are things such as someone learning to grow cells in bottles; or viruses in these bottles of cells; or finding out the chemical composition of the gene; or finding out how genetic material can make more of itself. Even these breakthroughs are rare, and many of us get excited about things of a much smaller magnitude. It is no small victory for a scientist to find out that something that we have believed to be true for a long time is not really true at all. This kind of science is not like building a bridge or a building. It comes closer to the remodeling of an old house; it is necessary to tear out the old before you can install the new. Sometimes whole new ways of thinking have to be promulgated in order to make a little bit of progress.

The discovery of antibiotics, which in one fell swoop cured a wide variety of diseases, has led people to believe that cancer may fall the same way. I suppose that it is possible, but it does not appear to me to be very likely; and one of the purposes of this book is to explain why. I don't want to hold back the march of progress, but only to point out that much more understanding will be needed in the absence of a "magic bullet." Ultimately, the acquisition of understanding has real value even if someone should accidentally stumble on "a cure." While we're waiting for miracles to happen, it is important that we find out what the best surgical treatment for breast cancer is, and what factors in the cell make one tumor spread and another not. These are only a few of the many problems which remain to be solved.

This book is really three books in one: One book (Parts I and II) is a discussion of cancer research; the second (Part III) is a discussion of human cancer diagnoses and treatment; and the third book (Part IV) is a critique of the way that government supports cancer research. While each part might conceivably be expanded into separate books, they are all interdependent. For example: it is necessary to understand what both cancer research and therapy are all about in order to evaluate the efficacy of government programs to "conquer cancer."

Three separate books call for three different approaches:

The first book (Parts I and II) on cancer research is written from a research biologist's point of view. Research scientists are generally interested in exploring the frontiers of human knowledge. Once a problem is solved, it ceases to be of any particular interest. Scientists are therefore more concerned with new questions rather than old answers (even if the answer is only a day old). Were I a reporter or a scholar instead of a scientist, the emphasis would be on the answers that have already been found—but I'm not, so my bias is in favor of spending more time on the unanswered question.

The second book (Part III) on human cancer is an attempt to explore the problems faced by someone who has cancer, or who has a loved one with the disease. It is fraught with recurrent feelings of my own inadequacies when faced with many of these unsolvable problems. I hope that it will be useful in helping people to cope with them. Those of us who have walked these paths before can, hopefully, contribute something to people faced with the same problems now. Since so much is unknown, and much of what we think we know will later be shown to be wrong, I have tried not to be too specific with "answers"; but have preferred to indicate directions and approaches that people can take. Each person must find his own solution to his own problems, and this section of the book might help him to do this. Furthermore, the specific answers that are eventually decided upon must be worked out in the total environment in which an individual finds himself; which includes his physician, his family, and so forth.

The third book (Part IV) on cancer politics is an attempt to change trends in the support of cancer research, which I consider to be detrimental to the basic aims of cancer research. I see the future support of cancer research as tending to favor large grandiose projects at the expense of the creative independent investigator. I do not think that crash programs to "cure cancer" are going to be effective; and in the process of supporting these large projects much of what is good in independent cancer research is being trampled underfoot. The aim of this section on cancer politics is reform.

Part I relates to all of the other parts; it attempts to explain some simple concepts which will give the reader a "place to hang his hat." These unifying concepts might lead people away from the dogmatic, one solution approach to cancer—and toward something that corresponds more closely with reality.

I have been told that cancer and humor do not mix. Cancer is a grim and serious business, and the addition of even small amounts of humor is likely to be offensive. War is also serious business, and it has produced cartoonists such as Bill Mauldin and authors such as Joseph Heller who have portrayed not only the grim, but the humorous side of war. It is because cancer is so grim that some humor should—indeed, must—be included.

Besides, a bit of humor helps to remind both scientists and physicians that they are, after all, fallible human beings—not gods.

Ira Pilgrim

Salt Lake City, Utah

Contents

THE TOPIC OF CANCER

PART I

WHAT IS CANCER?

A child said, *What is the grass?* fetching it to me with full hands, How could I answer the child? I do not know what it is any more than he.

Walt Whitman, "Song of Myself"

Cancer and Other Four Letter Words

Words like _ _ _ _ and _ _ _ _ and such,
Don't bother people half as much.

The word tumor is—or was—a Latin word meaning swollen or
enlarged. People used to talk about the tumor of pregnancy, or
the tumor of infection or inflammation. The word tumor has
been converted to a noun meaning an abnormal growth,
and all other uses have become taboo. We now refer to the
"enlargement of pregnancy" ("greatness" was a good word, but
it isn't used much any more); the "swelling of inflammation"—
even the tumor of the passionate penis has been bowdlerized to
"tumescent." Tumor is still occasionally used to refer to pregnancy, but only in unmarried ladies who go to out-of-town
hospitals to have their "tumors" removed.

Most tumors either reach a finite size and stop growing, or
grow very slowly. Warts or moles are, by definition, tumors, as
are many other harmless (benign) swellings. If a tumor continues to grow so that it threatens the life of the individual, it is
called malignant (*mal* means "bad"; *bene* means "good"). Malignant tumors are divided into several types according to the
tissues of the body from which they come.

The tissues of the body can be divided into three broad
categories: epithelium, connective tissue, and nervous tissue.

Epithelium (epi = on, thelium = nipple—a word that now has a much broader meaning) is the tissue that covers the body surfaces, and everything that is derived from it or looks like it. The lining of your skin is epithelium, as is the lining of your mouth and intestine. Most of what makes up a piece of liver is epithelium, and a good part of what the kidney is composed of is also epithelium. The connective tissues include bone, muscle, and the cells and fibers that hold almost everything together (connective tissue proper). Steak consists largely of muscle, as does the heart. Leather is tanned connective tissue. The gristle in the meat you eat is also connective tissue. Nervous tissue is just called nervous tissue, which makes it one of the few medical terms that anyone can understand. Those malignant tumors derived from epithelium are called cancers or carcinomas. Those coming from connective tissue, bone, muscle, and other supportive tissues are called sarcomas (flesh tumors). Popular usage has made the word cancer synonymous with "malignant tumor" and I will use it in that way. Purists may be disconcerted when I talk about cancer of the blood cells or cancer of the bone, but (tough) that's the nature of language (as noted above, what once was "on the nipple" now also refers to the cells of the kidney, the liver, the skin, the adrenal gland, and so on). Tumors of nervous tissue are simply called "nerve tumors" (neuromas).

This division of tumors into good (benign) and bad (malignant) is okay as far as it goes, but it doesn't go very far. There are bad tumors that are very bad, some that are not so bad, and many that might be bad if not removed. There are also some "good" tumors that are very bad if they are in the wrong place and "good" tumors that can become bad. There is even the rare "bad" tumor that turns over a new leaf.

Sometimes cells from a tumor that arose in one part of the body end up in another part and proceed to grow. A tumor of the breast can end up growing in the bone; a tumor of the lung can end up in the brain; or a tumor of the skin can end up in the lung. When this happens it is called metastasis. Some tumors metastasize readily, and some do not. It is obvious that cutting off a skin tumor may not help much if it's already growing in the lung as well as in the skin. The really bad tumors, therefore, do a lot of metastasizing. Why some tumors do this and others don't is poorly understood, and will be discussed in more detail later on.

This book is about tumors and cancers and malignant and benign and metastasis and a whole mess of words that terrify human beings. It is strange that the words "cancer" and "malignant" terrify people far beyond the actual dangers posed by the diseases that they represent. Cancer is no more terrible than many other ways of dying such as automobile accidents, heart disease, strokes, and a wide variety of terrible things which happen to people. It is as if the word *cancer* has become the scapegoat of all of our fears, so that people may feel that if they do not have cancer, they are healthy; and if they do have cancer that they are doomed. Nothing can be further from the truth. There are worse ways of dying than of cancer; and very many people that have cancer are cured and go on to lead full productive lives—only to eventually die of something else. The word *cancer* has been known to kill: people who thought they were doomed have taken their own lives rather than submit to what they believed to be a large amount of suffering. Words can kill; and it is one of the purposes of this book to deliver people from the terror of the words so that the disease itself can be approached in a rational and meaningful way. I will try to explain what these words mean and what we do and don't understand about this biological process called cancer.

Anything Grows

Considering how many fools can calculate, it is surprising that it should be thought either a difficult or a tedious task for any other fool to learn how to master the same tricks.

Some calculus tricks are quite easy. Some are enormously difficult. The fools who write the textbooks of advanced mathematics—and they are mostly clever fools—seldom take the trouble to show you how easy the easy calculations are. On the contrary, they seem to desire to impress you with their tremendous cleverness by going about it in the most difficult way.

Being myself a remarkably stupid fellow, I have had to unteach myself the difficulties, and now beg to present to my fellow fools the parts that are not hard. Master these thoroughly, and the rest will follow. WHAT ONE FOOL CAN DO, ANOTHER CAN.

Silvanus P. Thompson *

Mathematics is not the only subject where people start with the more difficult concepts first and then work their way back to the simpler ones. People being introduced to the subject of cancer are first confronted with the complex concepts, and often never get near the simpler ones. The virus theory of cancer, or what cancers look like under the microscope or how they spread, is extremely complicated. In contrast, an overview of the dynamics of growth can be fairly simple.

It is much simpler to think of things in a frozen static state

* Silvanus P. Thompson, *Calculus Made Easy* (London: Macmillan & Co., 1961).

than to think of them in motion. People (including a majority of cancer biologists) prefer to think of things in discrete stages because their minds can handle static concepts more easily. No one has any particular difficulty with the concept of an automobile moving at a rate of speed, or of someone running at 12 miles per hour, yet we prefer to freeze time by saying that "he ran the mile in five minutes." One of the aims of the study of biology is to discover what "reality" is and isn't—and one thing that it isn't is things standing still. Living things are always in some form of motion and it is preferable, if possible, to deal with them while they are in motion.

As with speed and distance, it is important to distinguish between growth per se and growth rate. When we talk about rate we consider the factor of time. To say that a lump under the skin has grown from the size of a marble to the size of an orange is to describe growth. To say that it has grown from the size of a marble to the size of an orange in one month is to describe the growth rate. It is often hard for people to understand that while the growth rate may remain constant, the actual amount of growth (in mass) may appear to explode. The growth rate of the tumor may be slow and fairly constant. Yet, when it appears to go from the size of a marble to the size of an orange, or worse from the size of an orange to the size of a watermelon, people would ordinarily think that something has changed in the tumor; whereas in reality the only thing that has happened is that the tumor has continued to grow at the same logarithmic (exponential) rate. In other words, one cell divided into two at a constant rate resulting in growth by doubling (see the next chapter).

The general principle of growth is the same for tumors as it is for populations of people, genes, field mice, bacteria, or molecules. If you understand this general principle, you have the key to understanding what happens in cancer, population explosions, and some aspects of physical chemistry.

What is this principle around which cancer research and the study of growth can revolve? I'm almost ashamed to mention it, it's so simple and obvious. It is this: THE *RATE* AT WHICH SOMETHING GROWS IS EQUAL TO THE *RATE* AT

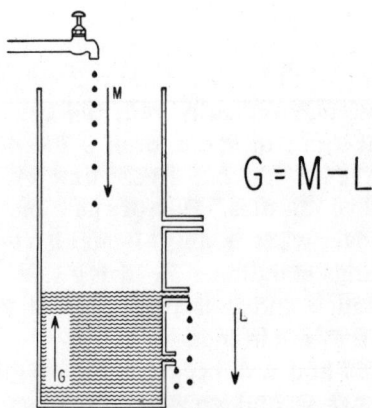

$$G = M - L$$

FIGURE I

WHICH THINGS GO IN MINUS THE *RATE* AT WHICH THINGS COME OUT. I have illustrated this by a little diagram (which I stole from the geneticist Curt Stern, who used it to describe genetic equilibrium).

This diagram shows that if you pour water into a pail that has holes in it, the rate at which the pail fills up is equal to the rate at which water goes in minus the rate at which water goes out. It won't do to let it stay like that; it's too pedestrian to merely verbally explain the obvious—we have to put it into mathematical form. The form is $G = M - L$. The G obviously means growth, or the rate at which the system grows (or the pail fills up). I have used M for the rate at which things go in because we are going to be dealing with an increase in cell numbers, which in most cases, is a function of cell division (mitosis). The letter L simply means loss, or cell loss, or the rate at which things go out of the system (or pail).

If you substitute human birth rate for M and human death rate for L, then G is the rate of population growth.

Observe that I am using the word growth to describe the end product. We all understand what growth means when we watch a child grow from 7 pounds to 150 pounds in a period of sixteen years. This "growth" that we observe is the result of cells being produced and cells being lost. When something "grows" or "shrinks" what we observe is the end product of an interaction between cells that are being produced and cells that are being lost.

It is important to remember that the growth rate has to be continuously greater than zero to have a cancer or a human population explosion. There are always short spurts of growth that either stop or regress later on. Our normal response to injury or infection involves temporary growth spurts. The total picture over a period of time is what is important, not momentary changes.

The principles of growth that cancers obey are no different from those for embryos, or cultures of bacteria, or populations of people or mice. These principles of growth are the same for both "normal" and "abnormal" growth. This is not surprising, since the border between normality and abnormality is an arbitrary line which divides the usual from the unusual or the desirable from the undesirable. The same kind of uncertainty that exists in separating the sane from the insane also exists in separating the normal tissues from the cancerous ones.

A many-celled organism always has things happening within it. Cells are always dividing, and cells are always being lost, usually at a phenomenal rate. Instead of a static state, we have what is called dynamic equilibrium. When you see that your left thumb has not gotten any bigger in the last several years, it does not mean that cells are not being reproduced, and discarded, but that the rate at which cells are being produced is the same as the rate at which cells are being lost. To prove this to your own satisfaction, just observe your fingernail. Unless you chop off the end of it, it grows. It is up to you to take care of the "LOSS" part of the equation with a pair of nail clippers.* The skin of your thumb, on the other hand, pretty well takes care of itself by obligingly sluffing off into the environment; it's called dandruff if clumps of cells sluff off on the top of your head. The magnitude of this skin cell loss can be appreciated by people who have had a limb in a cast for a

---

* You can calculate how fast the cells in your nail bed are dividing by measuring nail growth and knowing the height of the cell ($L = O$; therefore, $G = M$).

period of time. When the cast comes off, there are sheets of dead skin that have sluffed off and had no place to go.

We could try to solve the dandruff problem in the manner of the Hiawatha parody, "with the skin he made him mittens—and he put the fur side inside and he put the skin side outside." You can get away from this with dead skin—but with live skin the cells continue to divide, continue to sluff off—only they have no place to go and we have what is called a cyst, which continues to grow until it is either removed or breaks through to the outside and spills its contents. This cyst looks like a tumor from the outside, but differs from one because there is little or no real increase in the number of living cells. The thing that increases the size of the cyst is the accumulation of dead cells and debris on the inside. This can cause trouble by pressing on things; and a cyst of the brain can be very serious. Ordinarily, however, cysts are just a nuisance to everyone but the surgeon, who can make part of his living by removing them.

We generally distinguish cysts from true tumors even though they superficially look the same. To be a true tumor, there has to be an increase in the number of live cells present that has to continue until there is a visible mass that hadn't ought to be there. For a tumor to be malignant, it has to continue to grow until it kills the person or the animal bearing it. Some physicians and scientists don't consider a tumor to be malignant if it just continues to grow, provided that it stays in the same place and the cells don't move into tissues and organs where they don't belong. It is easy to see that the tumor that stays in one place and can be removed from an individual (in much the same way that you can take a nut out of its shell) is not particularly dangerous, provided that it is removed. At the same time, any tumor that continues to grow can become a hazard by pressing on vital organs. A tumor that reaches a certain size and then stops growing, or grows at such a slow rate as to be barely perceptible and stays in one place, is clearly benign; and it may be irrelevant whether it is removed or not.

Certain types of cells, such as the white blood cells, whose normal behavior requires them to circulate in the body, automatically become killers if the total number of cells continues to increase. It is not necessary that they change their behavior and invade organs where they're not supposed to be—because they are supposed to be everywhere. When these cells continue to circulate in the blood stream, a condition is produced which is called leukemia (white blood). This will be discussed later.

A tumor that continues to grow and does not invade surrounding tissue or metastasize can be just as deadly as one that does if it is located in a vital area. Before the advent of chest surgery, any progressively growing tumor of the lung was fatal because it could not be removed, and would eventually crowd out the lung to the point where the individual bearing it could no longer breathe. The same thing is true of some tumors of the brain, in which the tumor cannot be reached without killing the individual bearing it. On the other hand, a tumor with the ability to spread is harmless if it can be removed before that spreading has actually occurred. This is very often the case with small tumors of the skin. As the words are used today, calling a tumor malignant or benign tells the individual bearing it very little about his future. The terms "curable and incurable" and the probabilities of a tumor being one or the other are far more relevant if you happen to be in the business of predicting the future, or if you happen to be the patient.

This way of looking at cancer as a continuing dynamic process instead of a static state is very useful when you try to understand what cancer is. In the chapters to come, I will point out how this concept of "cancer as a dynamic process" is related to predicting the future of cancer research with regard to the probability of finding a "cure."

This ability of cells to reproduce and to die is the very basis of life. Without cells being born there would, of course, be no life. Without cells continually dying there would be no room on our planet for new life. This potential to reproduce also keeps our skin and intestine intact by allowing the repair of injuries. Imagine what would happen if every cut or scrape or infection that we received in a lifetime didn't heal. These miracles, which we take for granted, are of the same fabric that cancers are made of. Ecologists speak of the balance between an animal species and its food supply. This ecological balance within the body is necessary for the well-being of an individual. If not enough cells are reproduced, then we are unable to repair an injury; and if too many cells are reproduced, we have a tumor. It is important to remember again, that not enough cells dying accomplishes the same end as having too many cells being born—again the concept of balance.

While the principle of growth is a very simple one, its actual application can be extremely difficult. There are many factors which determine how rapidly or how frequently cells divide, with the result that this process rarely remains constant. The same is true of cell loss, which is influenced by a large number of factors—not the least of which is the surgeon's knife. Sometimes, trying to apply this principle in an experiment can be like trying to thread a needle while riding a bucking horse.

Why Tumors Seem Wild

If one amoeba divides into two, and two divide into four, and so on; how come we are not up to our ears in amoebas?

It is an established fact that cells reproduce by dividing from one cell into two. This does not seem to be a very profound statement to be making in the atomic age, but it is the key to what follows. If one cell divides into two, and the two resulting cells divide into four, and the four resulting cells divide into eight, we have what is known as exponential (or logarithmic) growth. This form of growth by doubling can have some profound effects. I have drawn a little chart that shows what will happen if a single cell continues to double at the rate of one every 24 hours.

As you can see, nothing discernible happens for a while; but by 20 days, the single cell has grown to a mass the size of the head of a pin; by 30 days, it's the size of a small die (half of a pair of dice)—and after that, the mass of cells appears to explode, so that 10 days later (40 days after the start), it is a liter, 10 days after that it's a thousand liters (264 gallons) and by about 120 days (from a single cell) it's approximately the size of the earth.

This "explosion" in the size of a tumor (which is the simple consequence of a constant rate of cell division, and the fact that

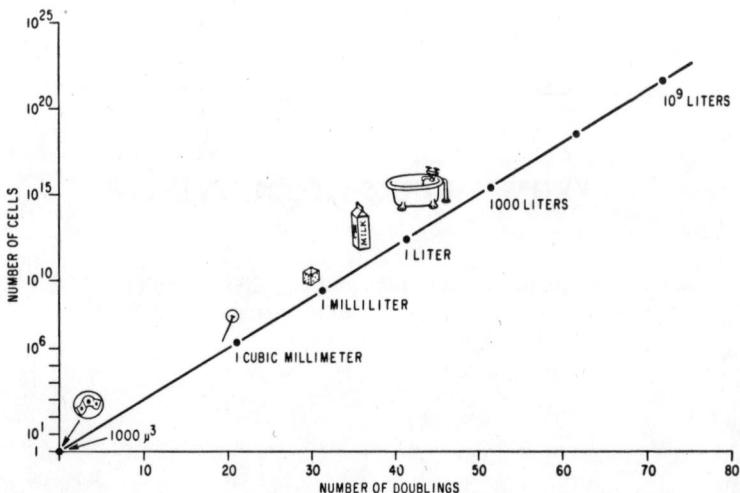

FIGURE 2

one cell divides into two) has led to the misconception that tumor cells divide faster as they get older. While this occasionally happens (tumor cells actually do start to divide faster), more often than not this "explosion" in size is simply due to the exponential way that tumors grow. This exponential growth pattern has also led to a number of other misconceptions, such as the idea that once a tumor is cut into, it grows faster. The cutting into it is probably coincidental, and if the tumor were not cut into, it would probably grow in the same way. In other words, most of this so-called tumor explosion can be accounted for by exponential growth—a consequence of the simple fact that one cell divides into two.

Early embryos grow exponentially, as do their organs. Obviously, this exponential growth doesn't last for very long. If an individual continued to grow at the same rate as he grew as an embryo the whole world could not contain him. What initiates the division of cells, and what stops them, is one of the great mysteries in biology. The answer is not known. There have been some interesting observations about what conditions are necessary to start and stop growth, but we still know little about the actual mechanisms.

We know, for example, that the potential for growth exists in most cells of the body. If you cut out a small piece of skin, the cells surrounding it divide and close up the hole. The same thing happens with connective tissue. If you take out a part of the liver, the rest of the liver will grow to achieve almost the same size as the original organ. The same thing is true of the adrenal gland and a number of other tissues. However, nerve cells apparently do not reproduce in the adult, nor do muscle cells (cancers of nerve and muscle cells are uncommon).

Michael Abercrombie found that cells grown in a culture dish will stop dividing when they form a layer that covers the bottom of the dish. If you cut out a wedge of cells, the adjacent cells will start dividing again to fill up the gap. We don't understand how the cells manage to know what to do.

There are feedback mechanisms which control the production of certain cells and keep the numbers of cells constant. For example, the loss of red blood cells due to bleeding or disease results in the kidney secreting a hormone called erythropoietin, which stimulates the production of more red blood cells. There are other mechanisms being investigated which are concerned with regulating the numbers of white blood cells in the blood.

Our bodies must respond to a large number of different conditions. The skin has to respond to temperature, the adrenal to various stresses, the ovaries have to undergo cyclic change, the child has to grow up to a certain age and then stop, growing bones have to grow to a certain length after which they have to harden and develop in such a way as to provide the best possible resistance to physical stresses, and so on. The timetables for initiating these changes are all different. Even if we should find that the cell has a single mechanism for responding to demands for growth and reproduction, we can be reasonably sure that whatever triggers the response will be different for different cells and organs. What is more, there is ample evidence now that we can expect wide differences in response from individual to individual. An interesting example of this individuality can be found if we observe what happens to different strains of mice when their ovaries are removed—a condition which simulates what happens when the ovaries have their function reduced by old age.

There are different strains of mice which are so highly inbred that they are similar to identical twins. What inbreeding in mice has done is essentially to take one genetic constitution and multiply it into a strain. Members of the same strain can exchange skin and organ grafts without reacting against each other. The rates at which they develop specific kinds of tumors is also relatively constant.

Let us use female mice from three inbred strains; we can call them strains A,B,C.* If we take the ovaries out of mice of strain "A", we will find that all of the signs of sex hormone activity soon disappear. The uterus shrinks in size and the cells of the vagina show the distinctive signs of the absence of all of the sex hormones produced by the ovary.

If we do the same thing with strain "B", we get a slight reduction in size of the uterus, and the cells of the vagina change to indicate the absence of hormones; but by three months the uterus is back to normal size and the cells of the vagina show ample evidence of hormone stimulation. Some even show signs of the typical cyclic changes that characterize the mouse's sexual cycle. It can be shown that the adrenal gland is producing the hormones that we usually associate with the ovary and that it is doing this in response to the pituitary hormones that ordinarily also stimulate the ovary (the gonadotropins).

Strain "C" shows an even more fascinating response. It undergoes the same general changes as in strain "B"; only this time we find that not only does the adrenal cortex (the outer part of the gland) change its appearance and start producing sex hormones, but almost every animal will develop a cancer of the adrenal cortex within a year after the operation.

Robert Huseby found that the differences between these strains is not a difference in the hormones produced, nor in the animal in general; but it is a very specific difference in the cells of the adrenal cortex itself.

It is reasonable to suspect that these kinds of differences between individuals and between strains of animals are char-

* For aficionados of inbred mice, strain "A" represents C57BL, strain "B" is the C3H strain, and "C" is the CE strain.

acteristic of all living things, and probably occur in every organ in an animal. The discovery of a regulatory mechanism that appears to be ubiquitous is generally followed by someone finding an exception to the rule.

Cancers themselves are highly individual. Cancers that have arisen in individual mice of one strain should all be genetically identical. Yet, each cancer behaves quite differently, even though they look alike and are produced by the same virus. One tumor may grow very slowly, and another very rapidly. One tumor may remain in the same place, and the other metastasize very rapidly. A tumor can arise in an animal, and be transplanted from one animal to another animal of the same strain. In the course of transplantation it may suddenly start to grow at a more rapid rate, and it continues to grow at the accelerated rate.

We know that the growth of normal breast tissue can be accelerated or retarded by sex hormones. The same applies to tumors, except that this matter of individuality comes into play. This is true in tumors of both mice and people. The removal of the ovaries will slow down one tumor, and do nothing to another; the injection of hormones may accelerate one tumor and do nothing to another. One might say that breast tumors have personalities and respond in very different ways to different stimuli. What is the reason for this highly variable response? No one knows.

My first contact with the word cancer was a description which described cancer as consisting of "wildly growing cells." Compared to bacteria or embryos, they're pretty tame. Cancer cells often reproduce at much slower rates than the tissue from which they arose. Most tumors of the intestine have much slower cell division rates than the normal intestine. The "wildness" of tumors really relates—as it does with teenagers—to their not knowing their place. The tumors may no longer respond to the influences that tell them either when to stop growing or in which direction to grow, or to stay in one place and not move all over the body where they don't belong. In the same way, some breast tumor cells are very responsive to sex hormones, or the lack of them, and some pay no mind at all. This is, of course, a superficial similarity in the ways that everything responds—and it is a matter of taste whether you consider the similarities to be more important than the differences.

In the past many scientists have equated cell division with tumor growth. There are some tumor systems where this is true, but there are also many where it is not. In tumors of the intestine, the rate of cell division is generally slower than the rate of cell division in the normal intestine itself. The reason that these tumors are malignant is because the cells invade the "inside" of the animal instead of obligingly sluffing off into the lumen of the intestine (the word lumen is a way of referring to the empty space surrounded by the intestine, which enables us to avoid calling it the hole inside; the part of the hose through which the water goes is the lumen). In the case of cancer of the intestine, therefore, one of the major problems is that cell loss does not occur as it occurs in the normal intestine. This, coupled with the fact that the tumor cells refuse to remain in one place, makes these tumors pretty serious, even though the cell division rate is slower than the rate in a normal intestine.

Apparently, most tissues have the capacity to grow rapidly. The growth of connective tissue around bone following a fracture resembles a malignant bone tumor enough so that it could confuse a pathologist into diagnosing it as cancer if he didn't know that there was a fracture present. Fortunately, physicians don't generally send pieces of regenerating bone to pathologists. The rate at which tissue grows around a fracture is phenomenal. The same thing is true of injured skin or intestine. The ability to reproduce is inherent in all living cells. The mystery is why they don't continue to grow. If we could understand the mechanism that stops growth, maybe the growth of some tumors might be controlled.

Since we really don't know what makes normal skin cells divide when they've been injured, nor what makes connective tissue cells divide when they're injured, nor what makes bone regenerate, and a whole wide variety of normal processes, you can see that we're very poorly equipped to cope with the changes that occur in cancer.

Man as a Hole

If you think that the mouth and the intestines are simply an extension of our skin, sword swallowing doesn't seem quite so miraculous.

A very useful concept when we talk about cancer—or about animals in general—is to clarify what we mean by the words inside and outside. If you think of a donut, the hole is actually outside the donut, and all the dough is inside. In much the same way, our entire digestive tract (from head to tail) is outside, just as our skin is. All of the rest—the meat so to speak—is inside. All lining cells of the outside (epithelium) have some basic similarity, but undergo modifications depending upon their location and function. One of the major functions of our skin is to keep us from drying out; hence the relatively impermeable outer layer. The same cells on the inside of the mouth not only don't have to keep us dry, but have a distinct need to remain wet since their function is, in part, to lubricate food for its passage down the intestinal tract. Some of the cells are modified to form salivary glands which secrete copious quantities of lubricant (saliva). The esophagus, which passes from the mouth to the stomach, has a lining that is not too different from the inside of the mouth. The stomach and remaining part of the intestine have the function of digestion rather than abrasion-resistance, as does the skin, the inside of the mouth, and the esophagus. The same modifications that help to keep bacteria from invading the skin also work to keep bacteria from invading the wall of the intestine.

There are other parts of the body where the "outside" pushes tunnels into the organism, with the tunnels still retaining some of the characteristics of "outside." The ear canal is a good example, as is the urinary bladder, the vagina, the windpipe, and the lungs. The lining of the uterus (womb) in which the child develops is also outside and, like the kangaroo's pouch, supplies a warm environment in which babies can grow. The fertilization of the egg ordinarily occurs on the outside. The ovary itself is "inside," but it sheds the egg into the fallopian tube (which is outside) and is fertilized there. The embryo goes to the uterus and sets up light housekeeping. It is partly because the embryo is kept on the outside that the mother does not ordinarily immunologically reject the infant. While this failure of the rejection mechanism is generally true, it is by no means always true. The exceptions can cause considerable trouble, particularly for the infant, since it is not in a particularly good position to defend itself.

When some of the cells of the placenta which are supposed to be outside lose their sense of direction and invade the inside of the mother (a rare event), we have a highly malignant tumor called a choriocarcinoma. This concept of "inside" and "outside" is useful because, as long as tumors stay outside they are easy to get at, can be removed surgically, and (unless they are pretty large) don't cause much trouble. It is when tumor cells penetrate to the inside that a patient is in trouble. Tumors of cells that are normally on the inside, especially cells that normally move around on the inside, cause real trouble.

There are cells whose business it is to wander around the body. Most of these are cells involved in defending an animal against injury or the invasion of microorganisms from the outside. The first line of defense is a white blood cell called the neutrophil, which is the main constituent of pus; it is produced in bone marrow and circulates in the bloodstream. The cells that ordinarily circulate are cells that will no longer reproduce (divide); they are "end cells." Occasionally, the cells that give rise to these neutrophils (a whole family of cells that goes by the name of the myeloid series) proceed to multiply in a manner that is greater than the rate at which they are used. Whether they do this because they no longer respond to the feedback controls—or what the mechanism is—is unknown. When these myeloid cells multiply, they spill out of the bone marrow and, following their normal propensities, circulate in the blood. The condition produced is called myeloid leukemia, and it is a lethal disease.

The second line of defense against disease is a whole series of cells that are concerned with the manufacture of antibodies. The exact interrelationship of these cells is not too clearly understood, although a good deal of fruitful work is being performed in an attempt to understand it. The principal circulating cell is another white blood cell called the lymphocyte. This cell appears to be able to recognize very specific types of invaders and respond accordingly. The lymphocyte is ordinarily a very long-lived cell that circulates and recirculates in the bloodstream, apparently searching for any of the particular types of microorganism that will trigger it into doing its thing, which is to eventually manufacture antibodies against that organism (although when it does start to manufacture antibodies it undergoes a considerable amount of change and ends up as a cell called the plasma cell; nobody knows what happens to the plasma cell when its work is finished). When an animal produces lymphocytes far beyond what the animal can use, a condition called lymphatic leukemia is produced. Lymphocytes continue to behave in their usual manner and continue to circulate in the blood and, since there are too many of them, they really gum things up. There are some sedentary cells that look like lymphocytes, but do not circulate; and when these noncirculating cells are produced in excess we have a condition called lymphosarcoma (a solid, noncirculating tumor), as distinguished from leukemia.

Both lymphocytes and myeloid cells can reproduce at varying rates. When the numbers of cells increase very rapidly the condition is referred to as "acute leukemia." When they increase slowly the disease is referred to as "chronic leukemia."

There are other types of wandering cells (macrophages), which we will not discuss here. When they do become tumors, they continue to wander, and are almost invariably malignant. There is no way of surgically removing a tumor of wandering cells. All treatments have to be based on some form of differential killing, either with chemicals or radiation. The rapidity with which leukemia kills is a function of how rapidly it is growing, which in turn, may be a function of the magnitude or type of the change that has occurred in the cells.

Some cells spread in very specific ways. There is a tumor called Hodgkin's disease, which is a tumor of one or more of the cells that are concerned with chronic inflammation—the kind of inflammation that stays around for a long time and gets better or worse slowly. This tumor apparently picks very specific places to grow. Some tumor cells prefer to live in lymph nodes and some prefer to live in the spleen. In the early stages of this disease, the tumor may be confined to several very specific areas. When it overgrows its specific sites it spreads all over the body to all organs.

Cells of the skin or intestine (remember these are both on the "outside" of the organism) naturally divide at a very rapid rate. They have to, in order to keep pace with the number of cells that are continually being sluffed off. In order for these cells to produce a malignant tumor, it is not necessary that any change in their rate of cell division occur; but it is necessary that they, in some way, forget where they are supposed to be and decide that they want to live in the "inside" of the animal. Living in the inside of the animal and dividing at their naturally rapid rate will produce all sorts of problems. If, besides deciding that they want to live in the inside of the animal, they also develop the capacity to grow in places where they would ordinarily not do so, such as the lung, the individual bearing these cells is in real trouble.

We have talked about how important it is for cells that are on the outside of the animal to know enough to remain outside (i.e., not to invade the inside of the animal). These relationships are established fairly early in embryonic development, and one of the most interesting aspects of this is the question of what keeps the skin side outside and the inside inside.

Malcolm Steinberg at Princeton has taken large numbers of different types of embryonic cells and mixed them together. The loose cells aggregate into a ball, with one type of cell on the inside, and the other on the outside. He has found that cells behave in much the same way as oil droplets in water; there is a clear relationship as to which substance is inside and which substance is outside depending on their physical properties. He has developed a way of measuring cohesiveness of different types of cells grown in test tubes, and can predict on the basis of their cohesiveness what will happen when you mix two different types of cells together: which type of cell will find itself on the outside and which type of cell will find itself on the inside. This type of work performed on skin and skin tumors and their relationship to connective tissue may very well explain what types of changes are necessary in skin cells for them to develop the capacity to move into the inside of the animal.

The concept of an animal having an inside and an outside is useful because it defines one of the most important problems in differentiation. We all of us started as a single cell, and in the process of "differentiation" this single cell divided, not only into a large number of cells, but into cells of different kinds. These different kinds of cells come together in a particular arrangement according to information that is already in the cells (in their genes). All that I can do is marvel at the precision and order with which this is done. I cannot explain it—nor can anyone else. Science has done a superb job of finding out how things happen (this is the main accomplishment of experimental embryology to date), but we have discovered very little about why they happen.

PART II

WHAT WE DON'T KNOW ABOUT CANCER

It is almost an intrinsic part of our concept of science that we never know enough. At all times one could almost say: We can explain it all, but understand only very little.

Erwin Chargaff, "Preface to a Grammar of Biology"

Not Another Breakthrough?

A brilliant idea for an experiment is one that works out successfully; a silly idea is the one that doesn't work out. Both
may sound equally nonsensical when first proposed. A Sunday
morning experiment is one that the investigator is ashamed
to try out except on Sunday morning when everybody else
is absent from the laboratory and can't make fun of him.
There is no scientific basis for making a decision.

Harold L. Stewart, "The Cancer Investigator"
in *Cancer Research*

Whenever I see that a new discovery has been made in cancer,
either in the scientific literature or in the popular press, I
withhold my judgment about its validity until the discovery
has been confirmed by other scientists—because much of the
stuff that is published is probably wrong. The skepticism applies not only to works of the new investigator, but to the
work of many of the established scientists.

Every time that I am tempted to readily accept something
that someone else has published, I remember *Spiroptera
neoplastica*. That was the name of the parasitic worm in rats
that won Johannes Fibiger of Denmark the Nobel Prize in
Medicine and Physiology in 1926. He won it for showing that
stomach cancer in rats was caused by this roundworm. The
work could not be repeated by the many scientists who tried.
The Nobel Committee has been cautious ever since, and the
next Nobel Prizes for cancer studies were awarded forty years
later in 1966 to Charles B. Huggins and Francis Peyton Rous.

Both of these men did their significant work at least thirty years before the awarding of the Prize. Rous showed that a transmissible virus can cause cancer in birds, fifty-five years before being awarded the Nobel. Huggins (1936) successfully treated cancer of the prostate gland with castration and sex hormones.

I don't mean to snicker at Fibiger's work. He was an honest and brilliant scientist, Charles Oberling refers to his experiments as "among the most brilliant in all the domain of cancer research." Fibiger found one cage of rats with stomach cancer, and found worms inside the tumors. He painstakingly followed one clue after another, and was eventually able to reproduce the condition in rats using these worms. Unfortunately, the phenomenon that he reported was not a consistent one, and other people were subsequently unable to obtain the same kinds of results that Fibiger did. Apparently the conditions in his laboratory were just right; the animals were on the proper diet, and so on. The worms might well have been carrying a specific virus; an explanation proposed by A. Borrel at the time of Fibiger's discovery. Borrel's proposals were ignored. At the present time there is no evidence for a virus, nor any other explanation for Fibiger's observation. It is an excellent example of a scientist coming to the wrong conclusions from the correct data.

This is not an infrequent occurrence in the scientific world, but it is rare for most of the scientific community to go along with it. The converse of this mistake, drawing the correct conclusions from the wrong data, also occurs. The classic example of this is the work of Charles Edouard Brown-Sèquard, who practiced his art in the late nineteenth century. He is sometimes called the "Father of Endocrinology." He had a genius for drawing the correct conclusions from the wrong data. He concluded that the adrenal glands were necessary for life because dogs died when he removed them. They also died when he removed only one of the pair of adrenal glands: something that should not have occurred if his surgery had been better. (An animal can live just as well with one adrenal gland as it can with two.) He also fed water extracts of testicle to animals and to himself and concluded that they possessed masculinizing activity. He was, of course, quite right; the adrenals are necessary to life, and the testis has masculinizing activity—except that the hormones that produced this masculinizing effect don't dissolve in water; and what's more can not be absorbed through the intestine in any great degree; his extracts were, in fact, worthless.

A scientist's acceptance of new scientific discovery has to be tentative. He must always be prepared to change what he accepts and does not accept as new evidence is brought forth. I hope that the scientific part of this book will have some value beyond one or two years. I have, therefore, placed very little emphasis on the "brand new" breakthroughs but have tried to restrict myself to things that I consider to be reasonably well established. The "breakthroughs" that made the headlines in the last year or so may be very important or may be entirely trivial. There is no way of knowing until they have been tested and confirmed under a wide variety of conditions. I have, therefore, avoided discussing many of the "discoveries" that make headlines—they will keep.

We read periodically that some scientist has found "the cause of cancer." If it were true, and there were a single cause of cancer, then prevention might be a simple matter. Unfortunately, there are many causes; and we understand very little about any of them. Let us consider the possibilities.

1. We know that most cells are capable of division, and that as a consequence, tissues are capable of growth. It is therefore possible for the regulatory mechanisms of the animal to push the button that says "go." If a small pellet of stilbestrol (a synthetic female sex hormone) is placed under the skin of certain strains of guinea pig, the animal crops up with what appears to be cancer of the connective tissue (fibrosarcoma). If the pellet is removed, the tumors go away. Another case is that of the breast of the rat: When a pellet of female sex hormone is placed under the skin of some strains of rats, they develop what appears to be typical breast cancer. If the hormone is removed, the cancer goes away. There are some people who feel that these are not "true cancers." It would be impossible to tell the difference, in people, between tumors produced in this

way and tumors that occur as a consequence of some change in the "genetic information" of the cell. We can sometimes tell the difference in experimental animals by transplanting the tumors. If the tumor grows in the new host, then the cancerous change has been in the cell itself, rather than in the whole animal. It may be that this phenomenon of tumors produced by hormonal changes may be responsible for some of the so-called spontaneous or miraculous cures. There are well-documented cases of patients having cancers of various sorts which disappeared without any treatment whatsoever.

2. Tumors can be produced by changing the information in the cell. This can be done by affecting the information already there by means of an agent which changes it (mutation), or it can be done by adding new information. These mutational changes might possibly be brought about by radiation, or selection of variants, or chemicals, while the addition of information would be the consequence of the entrance of a virus.

Much of the work in cancer research is devoted to trying to understand these "informational" phenomena: and it is a very fruitful avenue of research at this time because of the explosion of our knowledge in the field of chemical genetics and our increased understanding of the way that the gene works.

It has been discovered that the information that enables a gene to make a human being is contained in a very simple code. There are four basic substances (adenine, thymine, guanine, and cytosine), the combinations of which provide all of the information that the gene has to have. How this code works is now the principal occupation of many scientists in the world. Molecular biologists are beginning to understand how abnormal genes are constructed and how they affect the individual bearing them. It is all very new and very exciting. It is also very intricate and its discussion should be left to someone who knows something about it. James Watson has written a clear book on the subject. It would be poetic justice if I did discuss the gene since Watson seems to have no hesitation about discussing cancer in his book.

3. Another way in which tumors can be formed is by a slight disorder in whatever regulatory mechanism keeps tissues

and organs at a constant size. As we discussed in an earlier chapter, there is an equilibrium established between birth and death of cells, and anything which disturbs that equilibrium in favor of an increased number of cells can result in a tumor. This is a very exciting area of investigation because, at the present time, virtually nothing is known about it. It has largely been the province of the experimental embryologist, and while much has been discovered, the great advances in this field are in the future.

4. It is generally a good policy when one breaks down a problem into various segments to leave one blank space and say that there may be other possibilities that we are not aware of. Category number four is this blank space.

So—whenever you read about someone finding "the cause of cancer," you can attribute it to the scientist's excess enthusiasm or the tendency of the news media to exaggerate or oversimplify.

There are molecular biologists who believe that unraveling the genetic code and being able to manipulate the gene is "the key" to life. Since the gene is the fundamental regulator of many of the things that happen, this statement is fundamentally true. But to believe that just because we understand gene action we will be able to understand life in general (including cancer) is not true. Understanding the fundamental processes is an excellent start in trying to understand everything that is happening—but it is only a start. It is only a start, because we have to deal with problems of different kinds at different levels. Let me explain: A simple analogy using the automobile might help: We have to understand the structure of steel in order to produce the kind and quality of steel that is required to build an automobile engine. We have to understand things about traffic flow, automobile speeds, areas of congestion, people's driving habits, and so forth in order to build safe highways. These are all interrelated—yet knowing the structure of steel or the physics of the internal combustion engine is not likely to help us much in the design of a national highway system. There are levels of study and levels of understanding. In biology these levels are often related to the physical size of the object being studied. A surgeon who has to remove a diseased gallbladder finds the structure of DNA to be useless to him in this endeavor. What he needs is a detailed knowledge of the anatomy of the area of the gallbladder.

About twenty years ago, I heard the mathematical biophysicist Nicolas Rashevski illustrate this point. As I remember it, he stated, "We know that everything in the world is the result of the action and interaction of atoms and molecules. It is therefore possible to reconstruct the boot shape of the Italian peninsula in terms of the action and interaction of molecules. Anyone who tried to do it is crazy."

There are many "worlds" and each has to be handled in its own peculiar way. There is the world of atoms (the province of nuclear physics), molecules (chemistry), genes (molecular genetics), the interior of the cell (cell biology), the cell, populations of cells, tissues, organs, organ systems (histology and physiology), the whole individual (medicine), populations of individuals (communities, nations, the world), the solar system, etc. While there is a considerable amount of interaction between people in adjacent fields, most scientists have little more than a *Reader's Digest* (*Scientific American*, if you wish) understanding of fields remote from their own. There is nothing wrong with either the *Reader's Digest* or the *Scientific American*, but it falls far short of the depth of knowledge that an expert needs. A molecular biologist has no reliable way of evaluating the truth of what a cancer pathologists writes in Scientific American any more than the cancer pathologist has any real yardstick for evaluating the discoveries of the molecular biologist. There is a limit to how much understanding a human being can acquire in a lifetime. We go by instinct; instinct which tells us that someone's writing is fundamentally honest—but there aren't many of us who have not been misled. Just as Napoleon led an army to destruction, there is no guarantee that the pronouncements of a Nobel laureate are true.

It is human nature for a scientist to believe that what he is doing is more important than what anybody else is doing. I suppose that it's all right to humor him, but we shouldn't take these chauvinistic pronouncements too seriously—nor should they be so frequently quoted in the press.

Statistics

There are three kinds of lies: lies, damned lies, and statistics.

Disraeli

The above epigram is related to the fact that statistics are often used to "sell things." People use statistics to document almost everything, with the same statistics being used to document opposing points of view. The number of examples of perversion of statistics to serve almost any purpose are legion. The statistician who deals with cancer is in a very different position. His gain is dependent on his being completely and totally honest. The result is that cancer statistics are fundamentally reliable, and any problems which might cause one to question their reliability are based, not upon the statistical methods, but on some of the difficulties encountered in obtaining accurate information.

When a scientist does an experiment with 1,000 mice he knows that they are in their cages; and, if he is a good observer, he can tell what's happening to them. He knows the age of the mice when the experiment started, and when an animal dies he can record it with reasonable accuracy. This is not true with people. They move from one area to another and no one, at the present time, keeps close track of them except the Internal Revenue Service.

The state of Connecticut keeps very good records of the numbers of people with cancer, and the reliability of their diagnosis is extremely high. How accurate are the estimates of the total population in each age group? When Jack Benny says he's thirty-nine, can you believe it?

Using modern computers, it should be possible to keep track of every human being in the country from the time he is born. This would require that every time someone moved, married, or changed his name, this would have to be registered with the government. With social security numbers, this may be a real possibility at the present time. There is an understandable reluctance of the American public to submit to things that are generally associated with totalitarian governments. There is a basic conflict between the need for accurate information about the movements, activities, and diseases of people with what Americans consider to be the God-given right to get lost. If social security numbers were assigned at birth, and the various branches of the government, such as the Internal Revenue Service and the National Institutes of Health, talk to one another (a remote possibility), it might be possible to obtain some fairly reliable statistics about the makeup of the population of this country. As a scientist, I can see the desirability of knowing about population movements, and getting complete information about cancer statistics; but as a human being, I think that I might prefer to retain the privilege of getting lost if I wanted to. The thought of having to report my movements (which I do anyway in order to drive a car and earn money) is anathema. I wonder, though, whether it is worth retaining what little is left of the illusion that I am a free individual in a free country at the expense of knowing whether we are doing any good with regard to preventing or treating cancer.

To say that there are more cases or fewer cases of cancer tells us very little about what is really happening to a population of people. We may be having more cases of cancer simply because people are living longer; cancer being largely a disease of old age. We can get some information about what is really happening by looking at what the actuaries (these are the

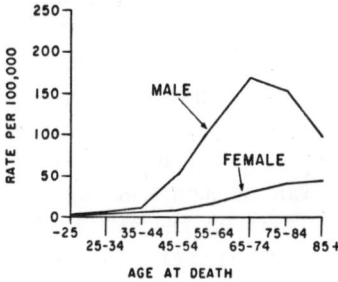

FIGURE 3

Average age specific death rates per 100,000 population for cancer of the lung, bronchus, and trachea, males and females, Connecticut 1949–1955.

people who predict the chances of your dying tomorrow) call the "age specific death rate." This tells you what percentage of a population at any particular age is dying of a particular disease —in our case, cancer.

Figure 3 gives the average age specific death rates per 100,000 population for cancer of the lung, bronchus, and trachea in Connecticut from 1949 to 1955, while Figure 4 does the same thing for 1956 to 1961; these are the cigarette-smoking associated cancers. If we look at Figure 3 and the line for males, you can see that this particular type of cancer starts

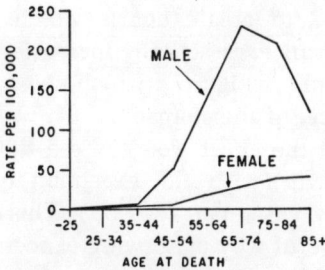

FIGURE 4

Average age specific death rates per 100,000 population for cancer of the lung, bronchus, and trachea, males and females, Connecticut 1956–1961.

appearing after 30 and the rate goes up progressively so that the peak incidence is between 65 and 74. If we were dealing only with a smoking population, the incidence would continue to climb; the reason for the drop is probably that there are a number of people who live past 74 who do not smoke and are left over, while the smokers are dying early. Now, if we want to know whether the rate of occurrence of lung cancer is going up, we compare the 55 to 64 age group in Figure 3 and the same age group in Figure 4 and find that the incidence has gone up from about 115 to 150 when we compare the five-year period starting in 1949 and the one starting in 1956 in this age group. This is not too convincing by itself, but when we compare the 65 to 74 age group, we find that this groups' cancers have also gone up from about 170 to about 225 in the same five-year period. This is very convincing and clearly indicates that lung cancer in males has gone up considerably. Not much has happened as far as the females are concerned. This is probably a cultural difference, and the liberated woman who smokes is likely to develop as much lung cancer as men before too long.

Another way of looking at what is happening with regard to cancer is a figure called "the age-adjusted cancer rate," which adjusts the occurrence of cancer for the entire population and enables us to compare cancer rates in a total population from year to year. How good these estimates are is a matter of the ability of the actuary to obtain an accurate estimate of the whole population and their ages. The age-adjusted death rate is used to create charts which show whether a particular type of cancer is actually increasing or decreasing. A good example of this is Figure 5 which shows the age-adjusted death rate for cancer of the stomach.

If you look at the chart, you can see that the rate is continually going down (with the exception of 1952 where it peaked to about 42 cases per 100,000). This way of observing trends is a very useful way of viewing cancer statistics. As you see, the incidence of cancer of the stomach is going down. It is now almost half of what it was in 1949.

I might add that the group of cancers collectively referred to as leukemia continue to go up until 1961. After 1961, it appeared to start going down. This has been attributed to the

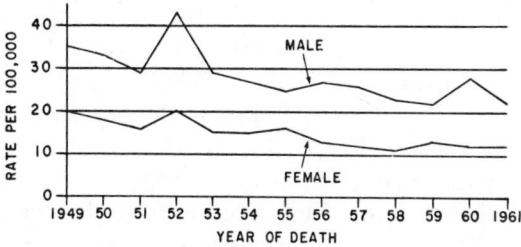

FIGURE 5

Age-adjusted death rates per 100,000 population
for cancer of the stomach,
males and females, Connecticut 1949–1961.

more prudent use of medical x-ray. This turndown in rate
started after 1943 in children under one year, in 1958 for people
fourteen years or over. The information being collected in the
next ten years should help clarify what is really happening.

You can, if you wish, read the age-adjusted incidence rates
in much the same way as you would read a stock market report.
For example, we can say that most cancers have remained unchanged. The averages (cancer at all sites) rose by about one-
third from 1935 to 1960. For the same period of time, stomach
cancer declined to about half of its 1935 level. In response to the
wide application of the Pap test, mortality due to cancer of the
uterus has also declined to about half of its 1935 level. Cancer of
the large intestine and pancreas showed a slight gain, cancer
of the rectum and esophagus about the same. In response to
increased tobacco sales, cancer of the respiratory system, particularly of the bronchus and lung, rose to about five times the
1935 levels in men, and showed a slight gain in women. Leukemia and related blood cell tumors about doubled since 1935.
The penny stocks (low incidence) such as cancer of the
prostate, urinary system, brain, central nervous system, and
thyriod all rose to about double the 1935 levels. Cancer of the
genital organs and breasts, after showing a dip between 1940
and 1945, came up and slightly surpassed the 1935 levels.*

* If you are interested in cancer statistics, the American Cancer
Society publishes a pamphlet annually called "Cancer Facts and Figures."
It is available for the asking.

We can interpret this as indicating that the cancer market is clearly bullish.

Statistics on human cancer can provide us with clues about what is causing cancer, and with the kinds of information that we need to enable us to determine whether the treatments that are being used are really effective. Human cancer statistics provided both the clues and the final evidence that showed that cigarette smoking caused lung cancer. It could not be determined any other way since, until very recently, no one was able to find a way to persuade a mouse to inhale a cigarette in the same way that human beings do. Attempts to produce cancer in mice with clouds of cigarette smoke failed. The statistical information on human lung cancer incidence correlated with tobacco smoking was sufficient to prove conclusively that cigarette smoking was the major factor in the increased incidence of lung cancer. The final bits of evidence were obtained by taking cigarette smoke condensates and painting them on the skin of mice and producing skin cancer rather than lung cancer, which showed that the chemicals in cigarette smoke could produce cancer. Someone has recently devised a way of piping cigarette smoke into the windpipe of dogs and is able to produce some of the changes that we see in people.

Scientists who obtain and use cancer statistics prefer to call themselves epidemiologists. It is reasonable to suspect that at least some of the clues about what is causing cancer will come from the work of these people. There have been a number of agents causing cancer in man that were discovered by this means. One of these is the chemical that causes cancer of the bladder in workers in the chemical industry. It was cancer statistics that showed that radiation produced leukemia in people.

We periodically read about "cancer houses," and the fact that an occasional cluster of the same kind of cancer may appear in a single location. We read in the newspapers about a group of young people who go to a particular high school all coming down with a relatively rare type of tumor. Is it cause and effect, or coincidence?

Finding a cluster of cases is an interesting clue, and it is possible that one of these clusters may yield some useful information. But by itself, finding a cluster of cases is of little value, and is really not worth publishing in the newspapers. The man who throws dice and wins twenty times in a row is doing something that is highly improbable (about one chance in a million); but this is no reason to assume that the dice are loaded—it might be a good idea to take a look at them, but you certainly can't accuse him of cheating. Improbable events happen all the time. The occurrence of improbable events is the basis for most accidents. The fact that four cars enter the same intersection at the same time is highly improbable, but once the crash has occurred, it becomes a certainty. The fact that once an event has occurred its probability is 100% is something that even escapes some statisticians. Most people are aware that a probability of 100% means certainty, now that the weather forecasts are being given in percentiles. When you hear the man on the radio say that the probability of precipitation is 20%, and you look out the window to see the rain pouring down, it should provoke at least a chuckle. We all know that when it's raining, the probability of it happening is 100%, and it makes little difference what the probability was before the rain started pouring down.

Chemical Carcinogenesis

> The fate of these people seems singularly hard; in their early infancy, they are most frequently treated with great brutality, and almost starved with cold and hunger; they are thrust up narrow, and sometimes hot chimnies, where they are bruised, burned, and almost suffocated; and when they get to puberty, become particularly liable to a most noisome, painful, and fatal disease.
>
> Percivall Pott's observations on cancer
> of the scrotum in chimney sweeps (1775)

The first reported "chemically induced" tumors were cancers of the scrotum in chimney sweeps in England. Why the favored site was the scrotum is a mystery. Presumably, boys in England, as here, were taught to wash their hands and face, and behind their ears. Fortunately, modern methods of cleaning chimnies, which do not involve using a small boy, were devised along with the use of cleaner fuels, so that chimney sweeps' cancer is a disease of the past.

Skin tumors were also well-known in workers in the tar industry. In 1915, two scientists, Katsusaburo Yamagiwa and Koichi Ichakawa, in Japan, were able to induce skin cancer in rabbits by repeated applications of tar. They were attempting to prove the "irritation hypothesis" of the cause of cancer. The irritation hypothesis of cancer grew out of the observation that cancers often arose at sites that were subject to repeated irritation. The hypothesis has not really been discarded, but has largely been supplanted by postulating the existence of viruses, specific chemicals, and other agents that might act at sites of irritation. No one has ever clarified the role of irritation in the production of cancer, so the hypothesis remains more or less in limbo. Everyone who has attempted to prove the irritation hypothesis has ended up finding something else. In the case of the induction of skin cancer in rabbits with tar, instead of proving the irritation hypothesis, Yamagiwa and Ichakawa opened up the whole new field of chemical carcinogenesis. It was soon discovered that there were specific chemicals that acted to cause cancer, apart from their ability to produce irritation. Irritation appears to play some role in the production of cancer, but we don't know what it is.

Following the discovery that cancer could be produced with coal tar, a good deal of work was done, largely in England, in an attempt to isolate the chemicals in the tar that were responsible for the skin cancers. A wide variety of compounds have since been isolated, and a good deal of very fine research has been devoted trying to understand how these chemicals act to produce tumors. There are now close to five hundred different chemical substances that have been shown to produce cancer. The implications with regard to our environment are obvious. Many of these compounds are the products of the incomplete combustion of hydrocarbons. Some of these anthracene-derived substances have been found in tobacco smoke, automobile exhausts, and in charcoal broiled steak.

Of particular interest are certain naphthylamine compounds which were discovered to produce cancer in the urinary bladder of workmen employed in the synthetic dye industry. These tumors often appear many many years after initial exposure to the carcinogen (cancer causer). It was very difficult to confirm the carcinogenic effect of these compounds on the bladder because most laboratory animals proved resistant (the exception to this was the dog, which reacts similarly to men).

Another interesting crystalline compound is urethane, which is rarely (but sometimes) injected as an anesthetic in man. It produced tumors of the lung in mice and, apparently, can also produce tumors of the liver and breast, and leukemia when it is administered soon after birth.

Unless something is done to change the trends, it appears that we will be continually exposed to more and more substances that have carcinogenic properties. Hopefully, we may be able to detect the activity of at least some of these before too much damage has been done.

The United States used to have a pretty high incidence of cancer of the stomach. This has plummeted to the point where this country is now at the bottom of the list with regard to mortality from cancer of the stomach. At the top of the list, in order, we find Japan, Finland, Austria; and joining the United States at the bottom of the list are Canada, Australia, and New Zealand. There has been some association of stomach cancer with populations that eat massive amounts of smoked fish and meats (it is important here to stress the word "massive"). With the price of smoked fish and meat being what it is, it isn't surprising that consumption has gone down in this country. These things have become luxury items rather than dietary staples. The fact that workers in the smoked fish and smoked meat industry who ate a considerable amount of smoked food have relatively high incidence of cancer of the intestines is no reason to stop eating ham or smoked fish, or charcoal broiling your hamburgers. We are talking about people who live on it. One would not expect the occasional consumption of active carcinogenic (cancer causing) chemicals to be particularly harmful to an individual any more than the occasional smoking of a cigarette would be (one exception to this bromide is with nitrosamines and bladder cancer, where one exposure is enough to cause cancer). However, I would certainly think twice about trying to survive exclusively on a diet of smoked oysters or smoked sturgeon, particularly when it's combined with rare vintage wines. Whoever said it was easy to be rich?

The smoked food explanation may be valid for areas of the world such as Finland, but it hardly explains the high incidence of stomach cancer in Japan, where they do not smoke their food, but salt it to preserve it.

Much has been done with the interaction of carcinogenic chemicals with other substances (cocarcinogens). A mouse can have its skin painted with a powerful carcinogenic hydrocarbon and not develop skin tumors. Months later, the skin can be painted with an irritant such as croton oil (which will not ordinarily produce cancer) and skin cancers appear. Mice that have been fed urethane (which produced lung tumors, but not skin cancer) develop skin cancer when their skin is later painted with croton oil.

There is a borderline between the chemical and the viral induction of cancer. This border was crossed when Francisco Duran-Reynals found that if you paint the skin of a mouse with methylcholanthrene (a powerful carcinogen) in doses that did not produce cancer, and subsequently innoculated the area with vaccinia (the virus used in vaccination against smallpox) cancers were produced. Perhaps it is similar phenomena to what occurs when a carcinogen and some other chemical (cocarcinogen) is used—or perhaps it is something entirely different. There are many theoretical explanations, but none have been proved.

Sometimes a chemical can be relatively harmless, but is converted into a carcinogen. An example of this is the nut of a variety of palm tree (cycas) which is used as a food in some Pacific islands. When fed to rats, the substance (cycasin) produces cancer of the kidney, brain, liver, and other organs. If the same compound is given to rats that do not have intestinal bacteria (germ-free rats), no tumors are produced. The bacteria produce an enzyme which converts the cycasin into another substance called aglycone, and it is this substance that produced the cancer.

Advocates of the virus theory attempt to explain chemical carcinogenesis by saying that the chemical activates a virus. However, in terms of what we know about the behavior of viruses to date, there is no real indication that this explanation has any validity.

No one has figured out how chemical substances produce cancer. There has been much superb research done in an attempt to explain their action. Several carefully thought-out theories have been proposed, and some are still hanging fire.

Three years ago a new dimension was added to the production of cancer with chemicals. This new dimension is the product of cancer in the children of mothers treated with a chemical during pregnancy. About twenty-five years ago the treatment fad for high-risk pregnancies (these are women who started bleeding early in pregnancy and presented the possibility that they might lose their child) was the administration of massive doses of stilbestrol (a relatively long-acting synthetic female hormone). Some twenty years after these hormones were administered eight young women, between 15 and 22 years of age, were found to have developed cancer of the vagina (at one hospital). Cancer of the vagina is a relatively rare form of cancer, and is almost unheard of in women in that age group. This led to a complete study in which the mothers of these children were interviewed in an attempt to find out what they had in common. It turned out, with only one exception, that the mothers of these young women with cancer of the vagina had been given stilbestrol early in their pregnancy. The physicians who did this study pointed out that the risk to a girl whose mother was treated with high-dose stilbestrol during pregnancy is a small one. The oldest female offspring of women treated with stilbestrol could not be over 28 years of age at this writing.

Perhaps someone will locate all of the offspring of women who have been given this hormone in their pregnancy and will find out what is happening to them. These cancers, if caught in time, appear to be curable. Like irradiation of the thymus in infants, which causes leukemia and cancer of the thyroid, this iatrogenic (physician produced) cancer marches on. It has been said that the road to hell is paved with good intentions. It is a pity that the hell is undergone not by those with the good intentions, but by their victims. The medical dark ages are not in the past, they are still with us.*

* To young ladies whose mothers took stilbestrol early in pregnancy: There is little need to be frightened, because the probability of your developing cancer of the vagina is very small. Considering the large number of women who took stilbestrol early in pregnancy, the number of cases of cancer of the vagina represents an extremely small fraction. There are, however, a few precautions that are worth taking that will insure that, if you are one of the few who will develop cancer, the cancer will not

Every time that an article appears in a newspaper or magazine that talks about cancer-causing substances in food many people panic. The question arises, Should I eat broiled meat because it contains known chemical carcinogens? By the same token, Should I go out in the sun, because I know that sunlight causes skin cancer?

Our world is full of cancer-causing substances, and there is no way that I know of to avoid all of them. The saving grace is that every chemical known to cause cancer has a dose effect; that is, the number of cancers increases with the dose of the substance. The same thing applies to ionizing radiation (see chapter "Radiation and Cancer.")

The only way that I know of to protect oneself against carcinogens in food is to vary diet so that you are not subsisting entirely on charcoal-broiled steaks, or entirely on smoked meat or fish. The human body will tolerate *small* doses of almost anything. (The risk of being killed in an automobile is considerably greater than the risk of dying of cancer of the intestine due to the ingestion of charcoal-broiled steaks.)

There seems to be little that can be done about cancerophobia—some of the victims of this disease would sooner commit suicide than run the risk of dying of cancer.

By the time you take away all of the cancer-causing substances, there is little in life to make it worth living. There is, however, little point in taking unnecessary risks. By unnecessary risks I would include fanatical sun worshiping, living on diet soft drinks, subsisting on a diet of smoked fish and meat, eating charcoal-broiled steaks for breakfast, lunch, and dinner, subjecting oneself to unnecessary x-rays, and, the most dangerous hazard of all, inhaling large amounts of cigarette smoke. It is also a good idea to do everything that can be done to keep our environment as free of carcinogens as we can.

---

be fatal. You should have an annual examination, including a Pap smear. Any vaginal bleeding occurring between menstrual periods should result in a very careful checkup. Any lumps in the wall of the vagina should be surgically removed. While there is not much data, the small bit of information that we have indicates that these cancers are curable by surgery.

A word should be said about what the statisticians call "competing risk." I can explain what is meant by competing risk by an example: It comes from a friend of mine who developed a sure method of winning at roulette. In the game of roulette, the probability of a ball falling in a black or a red slot is 50:50. In other words, the probability of winning is approximately the same as the probability of loosing in any turn of the wheel, provided that you play black or red. This fellow had a foolproof system: He would play black or red and he would play a dollar each time. If he won, he would keep the dollar and play another dollar. Suppose, however, that he lost. He would then play two dollars, and if he won, the extra dollar would pay for his previous loss and the next dollar would be a win. If he lost again, he would double up again and continue with the same procedure. Obviously, he couldn't lose, with one possible exception: A string of continuous losses could break him. This is where the competing risk comes in: If he goes broke before he wins the amount of money he has set out to win, then he has essentially lost the game. The probability of his going broke before he broke the bank is extremely high, particularly if the amount of capital he started out with was smaller than the amount of capital that the bank started out with.

Another example is a woman, age 80, who is surgically treated for breast cancer. The probability of her dying of something else before cancer reoccurs is extremely high. The same thing is true of cancer and heart disease in a heavy smoker. The chances of his dying of heart disease are reduced by the chances of dying of lung cancer before he gets heart disease and, in turn, the chances of his dying of lung cancer are reduced because of the chances of his dying of heart disease first.

I put this paragraph on competing risks into this chapter instead of the one on statistics because I think that it is more applicable here. Assuming that a small amount of any carcinogen would increase your chances of dying of cancer of the stomach, you have to consider the probability of your dying of something long before the effect of the carcinogen gets you. Examples of some relative risks would be as follows: (1) The probability in a heavy smoker of his dying of lung cancer is greater than the probability of his dying in an automobile accident. In a nonsmoker, the probability of dying in an automobile accident is greater than the probability of dying of lung cancer. (2) In a motorcycle rider, the probability of dying accidentally is greater than the probability of dying of cancer (if you have treatable leukemia you can reduce your chances of dying of leukemia by riding a motorcycle). (3) For a student airplane pilot the chances of his dying of cancer are less than his chances of dying accidentally. (4) The chances of someone living in Africa dying of cancer are less than the chances of someone living in the United States dying of cancer. (5) The chances of someone living in Africa dying of malaria are greater than the chances of someone living in the United States dying of malaria.

In other words, it is only if you intend to live forever that small doses of carcinogen are worth worrying about.

Tobacco Is a Deadly Weed!

Charles Lamb said 150 years or so ago:
"For thy sake, tobacco, I would do anything but die."
By the standards of many modern smokers, Mr. Lamb was a piker.

Everyone eventually stops smoking. Mother Nature—the most permissive of parents—sees to that. Those who smoke heaviest stop earliest.

Pat McGrady, *The Savage Cell*

To talk about whether cigarette smoking causes lung cancer is like beating a dead horse. Aside from a few cranks—who smoke and don't want to stop—and people who work for tobacco companies, there is no room for doubt that inhaling cigarette smoke is the single most potent carcinogen (cancer causer) for man. It accounts for more cancer and other deaths in this country than any agent known to cause disease in man. The case is so convincing that a jury would convict a man of murder on a fraction of the evidence.

At least 90 percent of all cases of lung cancer are due to cigarette smoking, and lung cancer kills more people in the United States than auto accidents. Your chances of dying before age 65 are about twice as great if you smoke cigarettes.

If you quit smoking for one year, it cuts the chances of your getting lung cancer by half. The reason that it only cuts it by half is that many people stop smoking because they have developed the symptoms of lung cancer. Once you have developed incurable lung cancer, it makes very little difference whether you continue smoking or not. The implication of the statistics is that, once the cancer has started, it makes little difference whether a person smokes or not. If the cancer has not started, the probability of it starting is reduced drastically when you stop smoking. It is so drastically reduced, that, if you haven't smoked for ten years, your chances of getting lung cancer is close to what it would have been if you had never smoked. It would be a mistake to assume that you could stop smoking at any time and, by so doing, reduce the chances of getting lung cancer to where it would have been if you had never smoked. If you wait too long, the lung cancer may have already started—not smoking from then on is not likely to do much good. I have discussed only the effect of cigarette smoking on the occurrence of lung cancer. I have not considered the fact that smoking has a deleterious effect on the heart. A heavy smoker may die of a heart attack as a consequence of his smoking long before he has a chance to develop lung cancer.

Smoke if you want to. It's your life, not mine. I quit over fifteen years ago after reading the statistics. Almost all of the scientists and physicians in cancer research have also quit; the ash trays at the meetings of the American Association for Cancer Research are unused.

Why is lung cancer largely a problem in the male? Don't women also smoke cigarettes? The most probable explanation for the lower lung cancer incidence in women is that, compared to men, there are few women who have smoked over a pack of cigarettes per day for over twenty years. It has been predicted that the rate of lung cancer in women will increase drastically in direct proportion to the number of women who become heavy smokers.

The cigarette companies are now directing their advertising at women. The modern woman is now supposed to have a cigarette in her hand—also stained teeth, tobacco breath, tobacco hair, lung cancer, emphysema, and heart disease. Apparently the tobacco companies would like to see one of the goals of woman's liberation be that of reducing female longevity to that of the male.

Why have I said nothing about pipe and cigar smoking?

Since the same carcinogenic substances are in all tobacco products, aren't they all equally dangerous? The substances in pipe and cigar smoke have the same chemicals and are, of course, equally dangerous. People who smoke pipes and cigars have an increased susceptibility to cancer of the lip and mouth as well as other parts of the digestive tract. If, however, we look at the death rates that are due to cancers caused by tobacco, we find that the cancers caused by pipes and cigars are a drop in the bucket compared to lung cancer; which is related to the habit of forcibly inhaling the smoke, which is ordinarily done only by cigarette smokers. As with most carcinogens, the frequency of cancer is a function of the amount of the carcinogen that reaches the site where the cancer will arise. When a cigarette smoker forcibly inhales the smoke, large amounts of carcinogen get to the lung tissue itself; while in the ordinary breathing of smoky air, much of the smoke is trapped in the bronchi (the upper air passages). The smoke particles are trapped in mucus which is later coughed up, swallowed, and excreted. The upper air passages as well as the skin, mouth, and intestines are equipped to provide a dead cell or mucus barrier to noxious substances, while the deeper parts of the lung are not.

While the Surgeon General fights to stop cigarette smoking, the Department of Agriculture and Congress promote it. The government, at the present time, is spending over sixty million dollars a year to support the tobacco industry. This is almost one-third of the 1970 budget for the National Cancer Institute, which includes support of the institute itself and most of the cancer research in the nation. In terms of its relative effectiveness, there is little question that the government spending has contributed considerably more toward causing cancer than it has toward curing or preventing it, since all of the efforts of cancer research have, to date, been unable to counteract the lethal effects of cigarette smoking. At the same time that we are trying to stop cigarette smoking in this country, the government spends $240,000 annually for advertising cigarettes abroad and 22.5 million dollars for tobacco donated under the Food for Peace program. Imagine that, poison donated under the Food for Peace program. Incidentally, the amount of money given to support the tobacco industry by the government (you and I, that is) is greater than the entire budget of the American Cancer Society.

Three years ago, I inquired of the Department of Agriculture concerning this expenditure to encourage smoking, and received a letter containing the following statement:

> During the 1970 calendar year 583 billion cigarettes were manufactured in the United States. The demand for tobacco products will continue even though confronted with health issues. Manufacturers will obviously strive to satisfy this demand and will obtain their tobacco requirements either from the United States producers or from suppliers of imported leaf. U.S. producers naturally feel they have every right to continue to earn their livelihood by producing tobacco to supply this demand.

This attitude was unchanged in 1973. If this attitude could be extended to heroin, who knows what economic advances this country might make. We might become the world's leading merchants of death.

The federal government has a vested interest in tobacco and is not inclined to do anything that will injure or antagonize the tobacco interests. An immense amount of public pressure could change this attitude, but the pressure would have to be very intense.

Taking cigarette commercials out of television and radio was an important step in reducing the effectiveness of cigarette advertising. Unfortunately, this elimination of TV and radio advertising was countered by an intensive campaign in newspapers, magazines, billboards, trains, and busses—all designed to encourage people to smoke cigarettes.

The warning inscription on the cigarette package that should have read (in large print) "Cigarette smoking causes lung cancer and heart disease" was watered down to read "The Surgeon General has determined that cigarette smoking is hazardous to your health." This says, in essence, "Big Daddy doesn't want you to smoke"—an irresistible challenge to a teen-ager. Besides, who is The Surgeon General? Does he still exist? What is his name? What does he know about cigarette smoking? The inscription on the package was a major victory for the tobacco companies because it relieved them of any legal liability for the people who are killed by tobacco.

The power of advertising is awesome. An advertising campaign could convince a very substantial number of people to eat arsenic for their health. The only way to counter it is a total ban on any form of tobacco advertising. It takes a substantial amount of my time countering advertisements that say it is good to smoke, alcohol is good for you, and if you are having trouble just take a couple of pills. If someone came here from an alien civilization, he would conclude that our society favors lung cancer, heart disease, alcoholism, and taking drugs.

The job of eradicating tobacco-caused disease apparently will not be done by government. I nominate the American Cancer Society and the American Heart Association, preferably working in concert. It will take an all-out campaign—this is one time where a WAR AGAINST CIGARETTES might work. There is a large amount of powerful and influential support for such a program. This support has not been mobilized and the campaigns to date have been puny and ineffective. The American Cancer Society directed conscientiously and single-mindedly toward the eradication of lung cancer could beat the tobacco companies. When Emerson Foote, a skilled advertising executive, joined the ACS I had high hopes, but apparently the consensus in the society was that it is better to "Fight Cancer with a Checkup and a Check." In my mind, there is considerable doubt as to whether these are effective weapons.

Tobacco products kill over 50,000 people each year from lung cancer alone (not to mention death from heart disease) and their pushers are still allowed to advertise in newspapers, on public trains, and next to public highways. If anything is to be done to prevent tobacco-caused disease, the first step should be the public refusing to tolerate the open merchandising of death and the hucksters attempt to convince the public that cigarettes are "good." Perhaps it's time to resort to vigilante tactics. The cigarette companies are winning and are using every dirty trick in the books. I suspect that if the true story of cigarette merchandising were ever told it would make Watergate sound like a rerun of Mary Poppins. The only thing that can stop these death merchants is massive public indignation. If every relative of everyone who died of lung cancer in the past ten years (a force of several million) took action, it would not be long before all cigarette advertising was stopped. Imagine every magazine and newspaper faced with a substantial loss of readers if they advertise cigarettes; or every cigarette poster with DEATH or LUNG CANCER or SLOW SUICIDE written on it in large letters.

My plan for the eradication of lung cancer is not as spectacular as an instantaneous chemical cure for cancer; however, it may work. The steps are as follows:

1. Boycott all newspapers and magazines that advertise cigarettes, and write them a letter telling them why they are being boycotted. Maybe the American Cancer Society might wish to provide a form which only has to be signed.

2. Insist that cigarette advertising be removed from all public places (it is offensive to contemporary moral standards) and cigarette vending machines be removed from all public buildings. Elective officials should be inundated with letters and phone calls urging them to do this. There is an old saying that "a politician may not know how to read, but he can count."

3. Sabotage cigarette ads: a felt-tipped marker does a good job. Simply write LUNG CANCER on all cigarette ads.

4. Publicize the image of cigarettes associated with derelicts and bums (the ACS uses this approach). Publicize the fact that super stars don't smoke.

5. Every time someone famous dies of lung cancer, publicize the fact that he was a heavy smoker. Edward R. Murrow was one of the most talented newsmen of our time. He was always seen on TV with a cigarette in his hand. He died at 57 years of age of lung cancer. A public awareness of why this man died before his time might have stopped some people from smoking. I stopped because the facts were frightening.

Communities have suppressed the advertising of nudity and pornography. To the best of my knowledge, nudity and pornography have never killed anyone. Cigarettes kill millions.

Radiation and Cancer

The rays called gamma and alpha and X
Have an effect quite different from sex.
They can change the genes,
And ruin the means,
Of making other human beans.

We are exposed to all kinds of radiation, ranging from infrared (heat) to cosmic rays. Radiation is a part of our environment, and nature has evolved a good deal of protection for all animals exposed to it. Our skin, and all of the glands associated with it, protects us against excessive heat, light, and so on. Some types of radiation can go clear through us without doing any harm.

The type of radiation that we are concerned with is "ionizing radiation," which is the kind that is capable of breaking molecules. These rays range from ultraviolet through a wide variety of atomic radiations.

Ultraviolet light can produce skin cancer in man and experimental animals. Human skin can tolerate a good deal of ultraviolet light, and there is a considerable variation in this tolerance from race to race—but, there are limits. The incidence of skin cancer is higher in fair-skinned people who are continually exposed to sunlight. This is especially true of farmers, and others whose occupations keep them in the sun for long periods of time. It occurs with twice the frequency in men as in women. There was a time when the standard of beauty in Europe and in this country was related to a white skin that was free of freckles and blemishes. During that era, physicians rarely saw cancer of the skin in a "beautiful woman." Our standards have changed, and the tan face and freckled nose are considered by many (including me) to be singularly attractive. The price of this attractiveness and the desire for a brown skin is an increased amount of skin cancer. People who receive a good deal of sun should be meticulous about having new skin lesions (sore that do not heal or tumors) removed before they grow to any appreciable size. Since the cure rate in skin cancer, if caught early, is high (over 95 percent) and the surgery is safe, there is little point in taking chances.

The radiation produced by x-ray machines, radioactive substances, and cosmic rays appears to act in a similar enough manner so that we can deal with them together. What I say about x-rays also applies to other forms of radioactivity.

The first people to use x-rays were not aware of its harmful effects. Many had fingers burned off by the effects of the rays, and a number of users developed cancer. There is no question that x-rays, or any other form of atomic radiation, will cause cancer, but there is a considerable void in our information about exactly how much it takes to produce it.

The incidence of leukemia in radiologists was higher than in other groups of physicians, and higher than in the general population. The induction of leukemia by radiation has been confirmed in animals and people.

Shrinking the thymus of newborn infants with x-ray was once a medical fad, and children so treated have an increased incidence of both thyroid cancer and leukemia. The incidence of leukemia in the survivors of the atomic bomb blast at Hiroshima and Nagasaki was very high.

There is a form of arthritis of the spine called ankylosing spondylitis which, in its early stages, is painful and results in the fusion (loss of flexibility) of the spine (the pain goes away when the fusion is complete). This condition was treated with large amounts of x-ray, particularly in England. The leukemia incidence in people so treated was high in comparison with untreated patients. Both ankylosing spondylitis and tuberculosis were treated with repeated injections of radium. Shortly after World War II about 2,000 German patients, children and adults, were given repeated injections of radium. By 1950 it was shown that the treatment was ineffective for tuberculosis and the use of radium for this disease was discontinued. Unfortunately, no one could *prove* that it was ineffective for ankylosing spondylitis so it is still being used. Charles W. Mays states that "at the present time [1973] about 100 new spondylitic patients are being injected with ^{224}Ra *each year* in Germany, because of the belief by some physicians that ^{224}Ra treatments may partially alleviate this disease." So far there have been 53 cases of bone cancer caused by this treatment *—what a way to cure arthritis!

The inhalation of radioactive substances can cause lung cancer. The deaths due to lung cancer in uranium miners in the unventilated mines of Europe appears to be about 50 percent. This may not be due entirely to the radiation because the incidence of lung cancer is ten times higher in American uranium miners who smoke cigarettes. The cigarette may account for the increase in the deaths due to lung cancer, in European miners of radioactive ores, from 25 percent in 1875–1912 to about 50 percent thereafter.

A certain amount of radiation is with us that we cannot possibly avoid; this is referred to as "background radiation." Some of it comes from outer space as cosmic rays, some from the radioactive elements in the soil, and some from isotopes in the air and water. One of the problems in evaluating the effects of low-dose radiation is that it is extremely difficult to experimentally achieve levels of radiation that would be below "background."

One of the scientific controversies with regard to the production of cancer by radiation is whether any amount of radiation will produce cancer, or if a certain minimum quantity must be applied. If a minimum number of rads (a unit of measurement of radiation) per individual is required to produce a cancer, then maintaining the amount of radiation exposure below that level will result in no radiation-induced cancers. If, on the other hand, effect is proportional to dose, halving the

---

* 47 cases from the tuberculosis treatment, 5 from treating ankylosing spondylitis, and 1 from other uses.

amount of radiation will halve the incidence of tumors. If X amount of radiation per person produced one cancer in 100 individuals, $\frac{1}{10}$ X would produce one tumor in 1,000 individuals; $\frac{1}{100}$ X would produce one tumor in 10,000 individuals, and 1/10,000 X would produce one cancer in 1,000,000 individuals. In other words, a small amount of radiation would produce a tumor in someone, if there is no threshold and the population is large enough.

With regard to the production of genetic changes with radiation, there appears to be no threshold. Any amount of radiation—no matter how small—can produce genetic change in at least one individual, if the population is large enough. With regard to some tumors (such as cancer of the bone) which require large amounts of radiation, there may be a "practical threshold." The amount of radiation required to produce one of these tumors in a very large population is so large that one would have to have an immense number of either experimental animals or people to produce even one tumor with a lesser amount of radiation.

The so-called bone seeking radioisotopes, such as strontium and radium, are able to deliver very large amounts of radiation to bone over a long period of time. The ladies who used to paint radium onto radium dial watches received very heavy exposure. They received this heavy exposure simply by wetting the tip of the paint brush that they used, with their tongues. Radioactive isotopes are extremely powerful (think of what 35 pounds of uranium^{235} did to Hiroshima). The amounts of strontium^{90} delivered to people by the fallout from atomic explosions has been considerable, when compared with the amount of that isotope that was present before the advent of the atomic age.

The argument has been presented that, since we do not know for sure whether this threshold exists, we cannot talk about possible "safe" levels and that a certain amount of environmental pollution with radiation can be justified. At the present time, it is possible to justify a certain amount of medical x-ray because we can equate it against its potential life-saving value. With regard to environmental pollution with long-lived radioisotopes, we have to consider the very important argument: What are the consequences of polluting our environment if there is no threshold? Once you turn off an x-ray machine, the radiation ceases—there is no way of turning off a radioactive isotope.

There is no doubt that any form of ionizing radiation can cause cancer. It will take a considerable amount of research to find out the relationship of the dose of radiation to the cancer incidence in animals, and we are probably unwilling to perform the corresponding experiments in human beings—at least I hope so. In terms of personal safety, I think that we have to proceed on the conservative assumption that there is no threshold and that any amount of radiation may produce tumors. On this basis, the risk, however small, of using radiation must be weighed against the benefits derived from it. The benefits of the medical use of x-ray outweighs the risk in many cases, contingent on the person using the x-ray taking precautions to make sure that as little x-ray as possible is used to achieve the necessary result, and that parts of the body that do not have to be exposed are not exposed. It is very hard to justify polluting our environment with long-lived radioactive isotopes.

The argument ranges between people who claim that there is no threshold and that any amount of exposure will do damage, and those who claim that there is a threshold and that we could tolerate a certain amount of increased radioactivity in our environment. The important question is not which side is correct, but what is the consequences of our making the wrong guess:

If we assume that there is no threshold, then the amount of radiation added to the environment must be kept at minimal levels. This means the complete cessation of atomic testing and the use of extreme caution when using atomic energy. The consequences of the cessation of atomic testing have to be measured in political, rather than biological, terms. If we assume that there is a threshold and continue to add long-lived radioactive isotopes to our environment, the consequences will be measured in more deformed children and both children and adults with cancer.

Embryos, Genes, and Cancer

The sperm and the egg unite to form a single cell. This cell proceeds to divide. The cells rearrange themselves until a fully formed animal is made. What causes this to happen is one of the great unsolved problems in biology.

The pathologists at the turn of the century were fascinated by the similarity of certain stages in the development of embryos to the appearance of certain cancers. There is even a tumor that consists of such a diversity of tissue types that one might consider it to be truly embryonic. It is called a teratoma. The cells that comprise this tumor are capable of becoming almost any tissue imaginable: nerve, muscle, connective tissue, blood, skin, and even teeth and hair. That a single cell is capable of doing this was shown by transplanting single cells, or groups of cells arising from a single cell, into animals; and finding that they still gave rise to the wide spectrum of tissues. This proved that one cell was capable of becoming all of these different tissues, rather than postulating that a whole bunch of different tumors arose at the same time—of course, fertilized eggs also give rise to different tissues. Teratomas can be artificially produced by transplanting the right piece of embryonic tissue into a mouse of the right strain—the right piece is the part of the embryo that eventually yields an ovary or testis.

An embryo is not a tumor because the cells do what they

are supposed to and the organs and tissues eventually stop growing. We know little more about what makes them stop, than we do about what makes them start again when they become tumors. The explanation of how cancers start does not begin with cancer, or even with the agent which triggers it; it starts with the egg. In order to understand the egg, we must go back and study the virus again; but not the virus as a destructive disease-causing agent, but as a basic life form. It is necessary to understand much more thoroughly than we do now how the egg unfolds to yield a complete individual; what the Germans called "developmental mechanics." While we are in the business of unraveling this, it is also important to understand the development of the fully formed individual; how his cells function, and how the entire organism functions.

As far as we know today, it is the genes that tell the cells what to do. A small amount of experimental evidence indicates that every cell in an individual has the same numbers of kinds of genes. This was done in frogs by taking the nucleus out of an egg and replacing it with the nucleus of an intestinal cell. At least some of the eggs that were handled in this way were developed into normal frogs. That kind of evidence is very convincing; and if it happens in frogs, it probably is basic and happens in everything else. The mechanism probably originated long before frogs or people were invented. If this is true, then every cell in our bodies has all of the information necessary to create another human being identical to us, but it doesn't do it. Not only that, but every cell has the capacity to become every other kind of cell; and if one cell becomes a tumor every other cell is capable of doing the same thing. None of these things happen—cells usually preserve their identity for the lifetime of an individual. No one knows *why* they do. If we are going to attempt to solve the cancer problem, here is one good place to start, among many others.

Every cell has a large number of genes. Of these, only a fraction are needed at any one time. The genes for making black pigment, for example, are not needed by cells in the liver. The genes that tell the cell to make mucus are not needed by skin cells, and so forth. There are a number of genes that probably function only in the embryo. Molecular geneticists talk about genes being turned on and being turned off. The precise way in which this mechanism functions is not known. Genes that were functioning in the cell could be turned off, or genes that were not functioning could be turned on. When this happens, the cell will behave differently from the way it did before the change.

Each one of us started as a single cell and, theoretically, all of our cells have the same numbers and kinds of genes. In practice, this is not true. All genes are subject to mutation (a change in the gene), and mutations occur continually. The mutation can consist of a small change in the gene itself, a rearrangement of the genes on the chromosomes, or the addition or loss of segments of chromosomes or of whole chromosomes. There is, therefore, a large amount of genetic variation in the cells of our bodies. Many mutations or chromosome changes are incompatible with the life of the cell, and the cell carrying the mutation simply dies. Others are of no consequence, the mutation is passed on from cell to cell, but does nothing to effect the cell's function for better or for worse. Still others may effect a cell only slightly. It may cause it to multiply a little faster or a little slower. If it causes it to multiply faster, then the cell will have a "selective advantage" over its neighbors and it won't be long before most of the cells in the area are of the same constitution as the mutated cell. If, on the other hand, the cell does not do quite as well, it will be at a· selective disadvantage and will probably be replaced by more successful cells. The same laws of natural selection that apply to populations of bacteria, fruit flies, animals, and plants also apply to populations of cells within the body of the single individual.

Genetic information can be added to a cell by the addition of a virus made up either of DNA or RNA. A DNA virus can incorporate into the cell and function as an additional gene, and an RNA virus is capable of producing changes in the information carried by the DNA.

Substances that inhibit cell division are found throughout

nature. We know that they exist, not because too many of them have been isolated, but because of their well-documented effects. Certain plants will prevent the growth of others, and it is now well established that the presence of certain bacteria will inhibit the growth of other bacteria. In bacteria, this mechanism is extremely useful to man and other animals harboring intestinal bacteria. Some of the normal bacteria which do not cause disease can inhibit the growth of disease causing bacteria. It ordinarily takes a very large dose of typhoid or paratyphoid organisms to produce an infection. In an animal without normal organisms this can be accomplished with only a few bacteria. This phenomenon of the inhibition of one organism by another goes by the name of antibiosis, and the substance that is isolated is called an antibiotic. If the antibiotics produced are not poisonous to man, then they become very useful drugs. You might remember, however, that bacteria knew about antibiotics long before we did. This phenomenon may have evolved along with other organisms with the result that all cells now produce some kind of substance that inhibits cell division around them. When the concentration of the cells becomes high enough, all cell division activity stops. These substances that inhibit cell division go by the name of chalones (pronounced *kal'ones*).

It is not really contradictory to say that a good deal of work has been done in an attempt to clarify the role of growth inhibitors and stimulators in a wide variety of cells, but the surface has barely been scratched.

If we are to understand cancer, we have to understand the basic laws of life—and nature keeps these well concealed. What we know about cancer today is less a function of what the people who have studied cancer have found out than it is a function of what has been discovered about biology in general. Every advance in science, particularly in biology and biological chemistry, has an application to the study of cancer. The domain of cancer research is, in fact, the domain of experimental biology.

Yes, Virginia, Viruses Do Cause Cancer

—and colds, and warts, and flu, and measles, and . . .

The best-known tumor virus in man is the virus that causes warts. This was first demonstrated to be infectious in 1894 and was clearly shown to be due to a virus in 1907, and there is still neither a cure nor a vaccine for it. More recent work has shown that it is a DNA virus—the virus itself is made up of the same type of material as our genes. Warts generally go away by themselves, and are also known to respond to almost any treatment.

S. L. Clemens describes several treatments for *verruca vulgaris* (warts). I have abstracted his 1875 paper as follows:

1. *Aqua spunkae* (spunk water): This reagent is collected in the forest and is an eluent of rotten stump. For the most effective therapeutic use it is necessary to apply it at midnight with the following injunction: "Barley-corn, barley-corn, Injun-meal shorts, Spunk water, spunk water, swaller these warts." Following the injunction it is necessary to leave the locale by taking eleven steps with your eyes shut and then turning around three times and walking home without speaking to anybody. "Because if you speak the charm's busted."

2. The Bean Method: "You take and split the bean, and

cut the wart so as to get some blood, and then you put the blood on one piece of the bean and take and dig a hole and bury it, 'bout midnight at the crossroads in the dark of the moon, and then you burn up the rest of the bean. You see, that piece that's got the blood on it will keep drawing and drawing, trying to fetch the other piece to it, and so that helps the blood to draw the wart, and pretty soon off she comes."

3. Dead Cat in Graveyard Method: "Why, you take your cat and go and get in the graveyard 'long about midnight when somebody that was wicked has been buried; and when it's midnight a devil will come, or maybe two or three, but you can't see 'em, you can only hear something like the wind, or maybe hear 'em talk; and when they're taking that feller away you heave your cat after 'em and say, 'Devil follow corpse, cat follow devil, warts follow cat, I'm done with ye!' " (This method has been attributed to H. Finn.)

Modern authorities feel that the *Aqua spunkae* should be applied two drops at a time for five days after meals. The injunction should be repeated at each application. With regard to the split bean method, only the bean *Phaseolus vulgaris* will do, and cross incisions should be used on the wart. With regard to the cat in the graveyard method, there is considerable disagreement as to whether the cat must be black, or whether it should be a male or a female.

There is little question about the efficacy of the above treatments provided, of course, that the patient has confidence in both the physician and the treatment.

So cancer can be caused by viruses—big deal! That statement is true, but it is only the first step in understanding what is happening. We know that colds, cold sores, influenza, measles, and so on are all "caused by viruses," but such a statement really asks more questions than it answers. The problem of virus-animal interaction is the problem of life itself, and is immensely intricate. Volumes have been written about it, and the field is still in its infancy. To hear some virologists talk it's "Plug virus into cell; wait 3.25 days; harvest virus—immunize mouse with virus; add virus-induced cancer cells—*voilà*—immunity, cure, Nobel Prize!"

The way that cancer viruses act is somewhat different from the way that disease viruses act. In virus disease, the virus attacks cells and either destroys or incapacitates them. When viruses cause cancer, they appear to do the opposite; instead of destroying the cells, they stimulate their continued survival.

Almost everyone is familiar with the lack of predictability of virus infections. The very same influenza virus can have no effect on one member of a family, make another member just slightly out of sorts, and make a third member of the family seriously ill.

Most of us harbor the virus of a cold sore (*Herpes simplex*), but when the disease erupts depends on many factors. Some people break out in cold sores under certain types of emotional stress and some break out in sores when they develop a fever. My particular bête noir is a spot on my chin that breaks out every time my face gets exposed to a lot of sunlight.

The same complex picture exists with the so-called oncogenic (cancer causing) viruses. There is a leukemia virus in some strains of mice that breaks out and causes leukemia in response to x-ray; another oncogenic virus, polyoma, doesn't ordinarily seem to do too much in most mice; but when it is souped-up in tissue culture it can cause large numbers of tumors in mice that were injected with it at birth (if the mice are injected with it as adults they develop a typical immunity and do not develop tumors).

There is a good deal of difference between different strains of mice as to whether they will grow or pass on a virus. Whether a particular virus that causes breast cancer in mice will grow depends upon the genetics of the animal it is injected into. If what is true between strains of mice also applies to man, then we can expect a wide individual variability in susceptibility to tumor viruses.

The more we know about viruses, the more complex the picture becomes. We now know that the breast cancer virus in mice is actually two agents—with one agent being passed in the egg, and the other in the mother's milk. The story about the discovery of the breast cancer virus (mammary tumor virus) in mice is an interesting one and bears repeating:

In the 1920s C. C. Little examined the pedigrees of mice reared and studied by Maude Slye. He found that the inheritance of breast cancer did not obey the usual laws of heredity. He and William Murray made crosses between mice of high cancer strains and low cancer strains. If the mother was of a high breast cancer strain and the father from a low breast cancer strain, the offspring developed a large amount of breast cancer—while if the father was of the high cancer strain and the mother from a low breast cancer strain, the offspring did not develop breast cancer. They theorized that there must be something that is passed to the young through the mother, but not through the father, and that it could not be a gene. This so-called extra-chromosomal factor could only be passed in one of three ways: through the egg, through the placenta, or through the mother's milk. The problem was too large for one person to solve, so it was split, and two possibilities were explored. Elizabeth Fekete explored the possibility of transmission through the egg, and in doing so invented ways of transplanting eggs from one mouse to another, and John Bittner tested the possible transmission through the milk. Bittner lucked out: The virus was transmitted through the milk of the mother—and what makes this even more phenomenal is that the virus is, to date, the only one that we know of that is transmitted through the milk of the mother. Bittner received the credit and the applause, and the other workers went back to the drawing boards. It is interesting that what is now called the "Bittner Virus" could very easily have been the Fekete virus. Another sidelight to this work is that based on discovery of this virus many people came out against breast feeding, stating that breast cancer could be wiped out if we could have one generation of bottle-fed babies. Unfortunately, there is no real evidence that a breast cancer virus is transmitted in human milk, and there is some evidence that early pregnancy and nursing might help to prevent breast cancer in the mother. It is a classic example of the danger of drawing conclusions before all of the information is in.

This "Bittner Virus" is one of the tumor viruses about which we have a good deal of information (perhaps more than any other tumor virus). An index of how complex the problem is can be gained from the following well-established information: The virus enters the mouse through the milk at the time that it is nursing. There is no apparent effect of this virus until the animal is about three months old, when a rare mouse will develop detectable changes in its mammary glands, and rarely a tumor. The changes are related to the hormones in the animal and can be induced by injecting hormones. The mouse has ten breasts—if you can call them that—and it's a matter of chance as to which breast will develop the first breast cancer. If the nipples are blocked on one side of the animal (an old experiment performed by Elizabeth Fekete at the Jackson Laboratory in Bar Harbor, Maine), more breast cancers develop on that side. Most of these tumors look about the same through the microscope, but the growth rate of each one is different. The tendency to metastasize to the lung is also different from one tumor to another. The age at which the tumors appear in the animals is different from one animal to another. The rate at which the tumors appear in the animals increases with the age of the animal. The transplantability of each tumor is different. If anyone can explain all of these things with a simple model, he will deserve the Nobel Prize, but no one has yet, and it seems unlikely that anyone ever will. If life were that simple, it would not have taken billions of years for it to evolve to its present state.

When a virus enters a cell and produces a tumor, it places its signature on the cell surface. Every cell of a virus-produced tumor has on its surface, and in its nucleus, a detectable protein characteristic for that particular virus. Tumors produced by chemicals are all individuals, and appear to have no such signature in common, indicating that they are not induced by one, or even two viruses. This doesn't bother me, but it is somewhat disconcerting to those who seek a single viral cause for cancer.

So, to say that "viruses cause cancer" is about as enlightening as saying that the ocean has fish in it—we are still little more than guessing about how viruses do what they do. There is lots left to understand. As for a cancer virus vaccine, we have to first find the cancer virus that we are going to vaccinate against, or else what is being done is little more than witchcraft.

So far, only one virus has been clearly implicated as causing a form of human cancer. This is the virus which causes Burkitt's lymphoma. Another virus reported as being related to a rare form of cancer is the virus of mumps. A high percentage of men who have developed tumors of the testicle were found to have had a history of mumps infection of the testicle. A prospective study has never been done; in fact these findings have all but been ignored by the people working with viruses and tumors.

I scratch my wart while pondering the virus problem— with a cold sore on my lip and a running nose. All three of these viruses have been my intermittent companions for at least twenty years. Someday, one of the viruses may make friends with some of my cells; and then who knows what will happen?

Cancer Immunology

Nature can be explored on many levels; none is more or less profound, none is more or less correct, but they are different. Which one you choose depends upon inclination, talent, accident, but most of all, unfortunately, upon fashion.

Erwin Chargaff, "Preface to a Grammar of Biology"

The science of immunology has its roots in attempts to understand how animals resist the invasion of bacteria. The study of man's resistance to infection appeared to become obsolete with the discovery of the sulfa drugs and antibiotics. What difference did antibodies make, if you could kill disease germs with antibiotics? It didn't take long before we found out that the killing of germs was only one part of the problem of resistance to disease. Furthermore, there are no antibiotics against viruses.

The discovery of human blood groups and the feasibility of transfusion opened up another field of immunology: the immunology of transplantation. Recently, there has been an increased interest in transplantation research. The technical (surgical) difficulties in transplanting organs have been pretty well surmounted, but most heart transplant patients have died, because no one has found a way of preventing the body from "rejecting" the "foreign" heart. At the present time, immunologic problems are the concern of some of the best minds in research. They are attacking the problem of how the body knows friend from enemy (self-recognition), the chemical structure of antibodies, the genetics of transplantation, and which cells of the body do what—and how (cellular immunology). Immunology has also fallen into the hands of the therapists.

One of the exciting problems in immunology is the problem of "self-recognition." We know that adult animals will "attack" bacteria, egg albumin, and all sorts of foreign substances that get to the inside of the animal. It does not attack its own cells under ordinary conditions. We know that cancer cells are also an animal's own cells, but there are some who claim that they are different enough to be recognized as foreign. There is some evidence for this: for one thing, certain tumors show microscopic evidence of an immune reaction around the tumors, and animals sometimes have antibodies against their own tumor cells. Unfortunately, this difference is usually not great enough to destroy the tumor. If it were, the tumor would not be there in the first place. If a tumor can outwit chemicals, radiation, and a host of other regulatory mechanisms, it can also outwit the immune system—and it does.

It has been known for a long time that an animal does react in some way against its tumors. In the last ten years, cancer immunologists have discovered that tumors induced by viruses have characteristics that are attributable to the virus that caused the tumor. A virus called polyoma will induce all sorts of tumors if it is injected into newborn animals. If the virus is injected into adult animals, the animal responds by producing antibodies against the virus in the same way as it does to any disease agent; and tumors are not produced. If two sets of animals of the same age and the same strain are injected with a tumor that has been produced by polyoma, it takes a hundred times as many tumor cells to get the tumor to "take" (to establish in the animals, and start to grow) in an animal that has antipolyoma antibodies than in one that is not immune. Antibodies against polyoma virus, which have been tagged with a fluorescent dye so that they can be seen, will attach themselves to the surface of the cells of any tumor that has been produced by polyoma virus.

Ten years ago, before cancer immunology became popular, an experimental therapist injected some of his patient's cancer into animals and produced antibodies against the cancer. The antibodies were concentrated and were injected into the patient's cancer. Sure enough, they attacked it and destroyed parts of it—the patient died. Antibodies can be used in much the same way as any other lethal chemical or x-ray or knife. The same problems exist with the use of antibodies that exist with the use of other agents, and most just don't work very well. One of the reasons that they don't work is that the tumor cells themselves have already escaped from whatever immunologic mechanisms the animal had, and the tumor cells also have the adaptive capacity to outwit most challenges. It might someday be possible to use an animal's own immune mechanism to fight a tumor, but it has not been effectively used to date in man.

With the exception of identical twins, every individual mouse or individual human is different from its fellows. These differences are genetically determined by a number of genes which result in a large number of possible genetic combinations. In the early days of cancer research, rare tumors were discovered which could be transplanted from one mouse to another or one rabbit to another; that is, they were able to cross the immune barriers between individuals. The differences between the tumor and the animal in which it was implanted still existed, but the tumor was able to kill the host before it could mount adequate immunological defenses which might, in turn, kill the tumor. When such tumors were treated by almost any means (surgery, chemicals, x-ray), the animal was cured of the tumor. Scientists were curing cancer right and left; and by using this type of artificial system they are still "curing cancer."

By the 1930s, enough strains of "inbred" mice had been produced to allow the transplantation of cancers to have some real meaning. Inbred mice are produced by mating a single brother-sister pair, and doing the same thing with their offspring. When this has been done for many generations, the result is a "strain" of mice in which all animals have the same genetic makeup. With an inbred strain of animals, it is possible to transplant skin, tumors, tissues, and organs from one animal to another within the strain, without engendering any immunologic reaction at all. Tumors have been kept alive for long periods of time by transplanting them from one mouse to another within the same strain. In these systems, the immunologic differences between the tumor and the animal are so weak that they can only be detected by very delicate quantitative technics and the "rejection" of a tumor transplant will occur only if a very small amount of tumor is inoculated.

The problems that are being tackled by immunologists may have a profound bearing on our understanding of cancer, disease, and graft rejection. Some of these are the following:

1. How does a cell recognize a substance, or cell, or microorganism as foreign?—in other words, how can an animal distinguish friend from enemy?

2. What is the relationship of the chemistry of antibody to the chemistry of the substance (antigen) that induced the formation of the antibody?

3. There are a number of different types of cells involved in the immune reaction: which cell does what, and how?

In 1964, Barbara Jacobs, at the American Medical Center in Denver, was attempting to grow some transplantable mouse tumors in organ culture (this is a technique whereby a small piece of tissue can be maintained in a dish in as close to a natural state as is technically possible). In order to test whether her organ cultures were still alive, she implanted the tumor cultures into mice of the same strain that the tumor came from. If her cultures were still alive, they would grow in the mice. A new technician implanted the cultures into mice of the wrong strain. Ordinarily, when such a mistake is made, the mice are discarded because—as every biologist knows—the transplants will be rejected and the tissue destroyed. Dr. Jacobs kept the animals. Much to her surprise, the tumors were not destroyed, but grew. Not only did they grow in a foreign strain, but when they were transplanted to more mice of the same foreign strain, they continued to grow. Something had happened to the tumors that kept them from being rejected. Another mistake? Maybe the tumors were not what they were supposed to be. No, because when these tumors were transplanted back into the original strain from which they had originated, they also grew. After the tumor had been grown in its original strain it "relearned the rules of transplantation" and could not be successfully transplanted into a foreign strain. Apparently the tumor had, in some unknown way, changed in organ culture so that it was able to violate the laws of transplantation. In the past nine years, a large number of experiments were performed which confirmed the original finding that tissues which are kept in organ culture change in some way so that they are not rejected by a foreign host. This may well be one of the most exciting discoveries in transplantation in our time; and it is a result of "cancer research." It might conceivably lead to our being able to transplant tissues and organs from one individual to another without their being rejected.

It is interesting that, to date, cancers have contributed more to our understanding of immunology than immunology has contributed to our understanding of cancer. Almost everything that is known about the chemistry of the antibody molecule has been obtained by studying the massive amounts of antibody that are produced by tumors of antibody forming cells (plasma cells) in man and the mouse. This is likely to also be true in the future, when tumors of other cells of the defense system are studied in detail. It would be interesting if cancer cells turned out to be the means by which scientists will obtain the knowledge that will allow them to transplant various organs across the barriers of individuality.

Everything You Want to Know About Sex and Cancer

by P

How does your sex life affect the chances of your getting cancer? Does the sensuous woman have more or less cancer than the celibate? And how about the man? Does circumcision help—and whom does it help? And what about orgasmic frequency?

There is very little need to answer these questions, because an increase or decrease in cancer is not likely to deter those who are enjoying sex nor encourage those who aren't. Nevertheless, with a "modern" book we have to have something about sex in it. I will deal with women and men separately because, although their sexual interaction is a thing in common, the types of cancer that are related to it are not.

Cancer of the breast appears to be influenced to some degree by reproduction. It has been known for some time that there is a relatively high incidence of breast cancer among nuns, and that marriage, having children, and nursing them appears to reduce the incidence. Since marriage, having children, and nursing are interrelated, it is very difficult to separate these factors. The early work suggested that long-term nursing reduced the incidence of breast cancer. This has never been substantiated, but we can still say that having children reduced the chances of getting breast cancer, and having children at a relatively early age appears to reduce the chances of getting breast cancer even more. It is also reasonably certain that having children and nursing them does not, as it does in mice, *increase* the incidence of breast cancer. In mice, the more pregnancy the more breast cancers. No one has ever satisfactorily explained this discrepancy.

Cancer of the uterine cervix has its highest incidence in prostitutes, and its lowest in nuns. That ought to tell you something.

You can't win, ladies, because what increases the risk of breast cancer decreases the risk of cancer of the uterine cervix: pregnancy reduces the incidence of cancer of the breast and increases the incidence of cancer of the cervix, while celibacy increases the incidence of cancer of the breast and reduces the incidence of cancer of the cervix. You might as well do what you enjoy, because in the long haul it makes little difference in terms of cancer risk.

Cancer of the penis is very rare in circumcised men and, interestingly enough, cancer of the uterine cervix has a very low incidence in women married to circumcised men. It has not been determined whether this represents a cause and effect relationship, or whether these observations are both due to a common factor, such as a high level of marital fidelity in wives of circumcised men.

The lowest incidence of cancer of the prostate is found in Japanese men. This has been attributed to the early and regular sex habits of the Japanese male—an orgasm a day keeps the urologist away. J. D. Fergusson says that "Exemption both from baldness and gout has been credited to eunuchs since Hippocratic times. More recently it was suggested that such individuals likewise enjoy immunity from prostatic cancer. Convincing proof of this is hard to obtain, but, as yet, no instances of the disease have been reported in such circumstances. From an experimental aspect, however, there is no doubt that in domestic animals subjected to early castration the prostate remains permanently underdeveloped, and it seems logical to suppose that a similar state in man might reduce any subsequent risk of malignant change. Despite this, it is obvious that prepubertal emasculation cannot be accounted an acceptable method of prophylaxis." Incidentally—castration is guaranteed to prevent cancer of the testicle.

There is a very very old joke that goes something like this: A salesman comes to the big city for a convention and is accosted at the train station by a woman who approaches him and says "I'm selling" and he replied "I'm buying," and they go off together. When he returns home, he finds that he has acquired gonorrhea. The following year, on his trip to the big city, he meets the same woman who says "I'm selling" and he replied "I'm buying" and again they go off together. On his return home, he finds that he has acquired syphilis. The following year he returns to the big city and meets the same woman at the station. She says "I'm selling," and he replies "What are you selling now, cancer?" Well, it looks as if this little dirty joke might well have been prophetic. A recent study, which has not been confirmed, indicates that people with cancer of the prostate tend to have had both venereal disease and a larger number of sexual partners than a control population that did not have cancer of the prostate. This appears to be a well-controlled study, but the samples are relatively small, and the conclusions drawn have to be tentative until the work has been repeated.

Some scientists have postulated that both cancer of the uterine cervix and cancer of the prostate might be caused by a herpes virus (a first cousin of the virus that causes cold sores). If this were so, one would expect some correlation between the national incidence of cancer of the uterus and the incidents of cancer of the prostate. There doesn't seem to be any such correlation with a country like Australia ranking in the top ten with cancer of the prostate and the bottom ten for cancer of the uterus; South Africa ranks first in cancer of the prostate and fifteenth in cancer of the uterus; while Venezuela ranks first in cancer of the uterus and twenty-fifth in incidence of cancer of the prostate. At the present time, I know of no satisfactory explanation for these conflicting findings. If a man wanted to play it safe, he would stick to one woman. He might have less fun, but he might also have considerably less trouble.

After reading this chapter, a woman told me that she thought that she would get neither cancer of the cervix nor cancer of the breast because she had had children at an early age, nursed them all, and had remained reasonably faithful to a series of circumcised men.

In summary, it appears as if people might reduce their chances of getting cancer a bit by having frequent sexual intercourse with the same partner and having children at a reasonably early age (now, doesn't that make you happy, Doctor Ruben?). To avoid cancer of the uterine cervix, celibacy can be recommended—but that is the only thing that it has to recommend it.

Two cancerophobes from South Boston
Used frequent sex as a precaution.
They indulged night and day,
In every known way,
And expired from chronic exhaustion.

Is Cancer Inherited?

My wife and I are both sterile. Is there any danger of passing
this on to our children?

Letter to government agency
Juliet Lowell, *Dear Sir*

We inherit a lot of characteristics from our parents that we
pretty well take for granted. We inherit arms, legs, livers,
and so on. Everything that we are is in some way influenced
by our heredity.

If an individual inherits a gene that causes death before
the age of five, we might say that this may be a cancer-
preventing gene. We may also inherit genes that contribute
to longevity, which might be considered as pro-cancer-and-
heart-disease genes, since cancer and heart disease are pri-
marily diseases of old age. The answer to the question about
whether susceptibility to cancer is influenced by heredity is
clearly a "yes."

But this is not really the question that most people are
deeply concerned about. The question asked is, "My mother
died of breast cancer; what are the chances of my doing the
same?"

What do we mean when we say that someone whose
parents had a particular form of disease has twice the chance
of developing that disease as people in the general population?
It simply means that those are the relative odds of developing

the disease, and does not take into consideration whether this difference is due to something genetic, a virus, or some common environmental factor. How much, if any, of these constitutional risks represent heredity and how much they represent other factors is not known. There is, for example, a slight increase in the risk of developing lung cancer in the relatives of people who have had lung cancer as compared to the controls. This difference is very small when it is compared with the difference between smokers and nonsmokers with regard to the same disease. There is a cultural tendency for the children of smokers to also smoke. With lung cancer, therefore, the environmental factor (smoking) far outweighs the genetic predisposition. If we consider just populations of nonsmokers, then there may be some inherited predisposition to develop lung cancer. We can't tell if this inherited predisposition is genetic or not; it might represent a common environmental factor such as urban air pollution. A very careful study would be needed to determine whether there actually was a hereditary predisposition to lung cancer apart from smoking, air pollution, and other known environmental carcinogens.

There are a few types of tumors where the mode of inheritance is known:

Von Recklinghausen's neurofibromatosis is a dominantly inherited condition which often results in skeletal deformity, and the presence of many skin tumors and tumors of nerves. Ordinarily these tumors are benign, but there is a tendency for people with this disease to sometimes develop neurogenic sarcomas (cancers of the cells of the nerve sheath). There are people with this condition who live to a relatively old age. A similarly inherited disease is acoustic neuroma, in which people develop nerve sheath tumors of the nerve responsible for hearing, and deafness often results.

Retinoblastoma is transmitted by dominant gene and results in the development of tumors of the retina of the eye. These tumors appear early in childhood and result in the death of the child unless the affected eye is removed.

Xeroderma pigmentosum is inherited as a recessive. This

hereditary disease is characterized by a peculiar form of skin pigmentation, and the development of cancer of the skin on exposure to sunlight. The mystery of how it happens may be on the verge of being solved. There is a mechanism within the normal cell that is able to repair damage to DNA. Since DNA is continually damaged in the skin by ultraviolet radiation, the presence of this mechanism is essential to the maintenance of the genetic integrity of the skin cells. People with *Xeroderma pigmentosum* do not have this repair enzyme and cannot repair the damage done to their skin cells by ultraviolet radiation.

There is an inherited condition called Gardner's syndrome, which predisposes people having this dominant gene to the development of polyps of the large intestine. These polyps often undergo cancerous change.

These diseases constitute an almost complete list of cancerous and precancerous conditions in which the hereditary factors have been clearly characterized. With other conditions in which a familial disposition exists, no one knows what that familial disposition is due to.

A woman with a close relative having had breast cancer has about two to three times the chance of developing the disease as does someone with no family history of breast cancer. To give us some perspective, it should be pointed out that a woman who has never born children has at least twice the risk of developing breast cancer as one who has. Therefore, a woman with no family history of breast cancer, who has had no children, has about the same chance of developing breast cancer as a woman with a family history of breast cancer who has had three or more children. Of course, a woman with no family history of breast cancer can cut the risk in half if she has three or more children.

Scientists have been working for forty years on the tendencies of different strains of mice to develop cancer. With few exceptions, we still do not understand why only certain strains of mice develop certain types of tumors. There are many differences between mice and people, and to extrapolate directly from mouse to man at this stage of the game would be folly. I mentioned in a previous chapter that there is a strain of mice in which 100 percent of the animals will develop adrenal cancers if the ovaries are removed. No one has reported an equivalent situation in women. There is a strain of animals in which all of the animals develop leukemia; but no one has reported a family in which the incidence is anywhere near that high. In short, we just do not know enough about the inheritance of cancer.

Just because you inherit a susceptibility to a particular form of cancer is nothing to lose sleep over. If you're not susceptible to a particular form of cancer, you would be susceptible to early death, or heart disease, or stroke—we all have to die of something, and an inherited susceptibility to cancer is not all bad.

It is natural that someone who has lost his parents to heart disease should worry about contracting heart disease, and that someone who has lost parents or close relatives to cancer should worry about dying of cancer. Taking reasonable precautions makes sense, but cancerophobia can sometimes be as debilitating a disease as cancer itself.

A rational approach to the problem involves the recognition of the fact that an increased probability of developing a particular type of cancer does not mean that one will develop it. You must also recognize that a twofold or threefold increase in the frequency of breast cancer still means that a woman will probably *not* develop breast cancer—but will die of something else. We must also recognize that a good part of the mortality due to cancer is related to the patient not being treated early enough. Taking all of these factors into consideration, a family history of a particular type of cancer is nothing to lose sleep over. Women whose relatives have had breast cancer should examine themselves at frequent intervals (as should women whose relatives have not developed breast cancer). The same principle applies for all other forms of cancer. I am reminded of a man who had a family history of stomach cancer. He drank to calm his fears, and died of cirrhosis of the liver.

Why Some Tumors Spread

If they only knew their place we wouldn't have all of this trouble!

If tumors would not spread (metastasize), the treatment of them would be considerably simplified—they could simply be cut out. It is their ability to spread which makes for their lethality.

Before discussing metastasis, I would like to make a distinction between tumors of white blood cells, such as lymphocytes, that normally wander, and when they become "tumors" continue to do the same, and cells of the skin, breast, intestine, and so on that have to undergo some change in their normal behavior to be malignant (i.e., they have to invade, and some will metastasize). I am going to confine the discussion in this chapter entirely to those cells that have to change their behavior (epithelium).

A popular misconception is that once the cells of a tumor enter the bloodstream, the individual bearing the tumor is doomed because they are bound to metastasize. Nothing could be further from the truth. An experiment that has been repeated over and over again (in mice) is one in which a breast cancer which does not ordinarily metastasize is massaged; the animal is killed and the lungs of the animal are looked at. Invariably, there are large numbers of cancer cells in the lung. In spite of this, other animals that are treated in the same way with the same tumor and are allowed to live do not develop metastasis. With some other lines of the same type of tumor, lung metastasis develops even if the tumor is not massaged. The body apparently has some mechanism for destroying cells that are not where they are supposed to be. An interesting experiment was done by Paul Weiss and Gert Andres in which they injected cells from one chick embryo into another chick embryo. They used pigmented cells from a pigmented chicken, which were injected into an albino (no pigment). They found that the pigment cells did not stay where they were not supposed to, and that some did settle down and grow where they were supposed to, in the skin. In other words, either the cells knew where they were going, or the body knew where they belonged, or both.

The work of Cameron Wallace on the metastasis of mouse breast cancer showed that some tumors metastasize readily while others do not. My own experience with mouse breast cancer confirms this. There is no way of telling by looking at the tumor under the microscope what it is going to do. If we take several lines of transplantable breast cancer which are microscopically indistinguishable and implant them into ten animals each, one transplanted line may show extensive metastasis in ten out of the ten animals, while other lines will show an occasional metastasis. The implication of this is that if a tumor is of the metastasizing kind, it will probably do so early in the game; and if it is the nonmetastasizing kind it takes a lot of tumor cells to get a metastasis started. Even a "nonmetastasizing" tumor will metastasize if given sufficient opportunity. It would be a mistake to draw extensive conclusions on the basis of this very meager evidence. There is a crying need for more research on what makes one tumor spread, and another stay in the same place. Until more evidence is forthcoming, it is necessary to use the surgeon's law of "When in doubt, cut it out," and add "cut it out while it is still small."

What is it then that makes tumors metastasize? There

is some indication that the ability to metastasize is in some way related to the ability of the tumor to grow in an extraordinary site. This is also related to how much of the tumor gets there. If you put enough tumor cells into a site, you will eventually get growth, even though the tumor would not ordinarily grow there. But this is not the ordinary state of affairs; what happens more often is that some tumors have the extraordinary ability to grow almost anywhere, even if small numbers of cells get there. There is also some evidence that certain tumors grow better in some organs than they do in others, and that it is not simply the trapping of cells that causes metastasis to appear.

The probability of a surgical cure for cancer is related to the ability of the tumor to metastasize. There are a few tumor types that are known to metastasize very readily, while some types do not. With most tumors, there is no sure way of telling by looking at them. This is certainly true with regard to breast tumors in mice. The only way that a scientist can find out if it will metastasize or not is to inoculate it into mice of the same strain, and see what happens. Your cancer specialist should be able to give you a better indication than I can of the odds that any particular type of human tumor will metastasize.

By the time a tumor is detected, some of the cells will probably have already spread. If the tumor is of the metastasizing kind, and only a few cells are able to produce a metastasis, then a surgical cure is unlikely. If, on the other hand, it is not of the readily metastasizing kind, then the surgical removal of the tumor will probably result in a complete cure. There is no way of telling by looking at the tumor under the microscope whether the tumor is of the metastasizing kind or not. Some odds can be given for different kinds of tumors, but they are only odds and tell you little about what will actually happen to an individual. The odds of being cured by an operation can be supplied by the physician—but they are only odds.

Suppose the tumor does not metastasize readily, what then? Again, the odds of the cells having left the tumor are pretty high, but the tumor cells have probably already been destroyed by the body. In this case, surgical removal of the tumor will probably have cured the patient. Suppose that the victim does not go to the doctor, and allows the tumor to grow to a large size? In this case, there is a very good possibility that the tumor (that does not readily metastasize) may metastasize because cells are being literally poured into the body. In this case, the probability of the cure will have been changed from almost certainty to something considerably less than that. Most tumors fall between these two extremes, so that the patient having the tumor can change the odds of a cure considerably by having the tumor removed at an early stage in its development. Considerable inroads in mortality due to cancer of the uterine cervix have been made by detecting abnormal growths before they have a chance to grow appreciably, or spread.

I would like to point out that no one has devised a way of determining, by looking at the tumor, whether it has spread or not. If tumors are detected at distant sites, then we know that it has spread. If they are not detected, then the only recourse is to wait and see if they appear. If they do not appear, they have not spread; and if they do appear then they have— it's as simple as that.

Is There an Answer?

Every speculation was once a guess, a hunch, a dream, a fancy, that the practical mind would dispose of at once. Imagination often flies in the face of logic, and soaring independently a discovery is made. All the work in library and laboratory never created a brilliant hypothesis. The hypothesis is the winged thought of the imaginative mind.

Harold L. Stewart, "The Cancer Investigator"

Several times a year, there is an article in the popular press that states that someone has just made a discovery about the cause of cancer. These announcements vary from modest reasonable claims to statements that imply that we now know the answer, and that the cure is not far behind. The fact is that we know more than we did five or ten years ago, and considerably more than we knew sixty or seventy years ago, but we are a long way from having solved the important basic problems. When we know what life is, then, perhaps, we may be able to understand what cancer is. It is natural that the cell biologist thinks that his discipline has the key that will unlock the door, as do the biochemist, the pathologist, and so on. It is natural, because scientists are also human beings; and being human beings they would like to think that what they are doing is of crucial importance. Unfortunately, none of this is true. No one can predict from which direction the major discoveries will come, and it is reasonable to expect that many discoveries will emanate from many quarters.

I have written Part II from the point of view of a scientist, which is quite different from that of a physician or a patient. The attitude of the scientist is sometimes hard to understand. Imagine a town being inundated by the lava flow from a neighboring volcano, and while everyone else is picking up their belongings and running as fast as they can, the scientist stands there with his notebook and camera recording the entire process. It is just this kind of detachment that makes for good science. Discoveries are made because a scientist looked at something in a way that is different from the way the rest of mankind looks at things.

I am in cancer research because of some personal events in my own life. I found out very early in the game that in order to be a good scientist it is necessary that I either approach subjects that I am not emotionally involved in, or figure out some way of short-circuiting that emotional element so that it doesn't get in the way (which may well be impossible). I find that I can make more headway if I approach the problem of life in general, rather than the problem of cancer as a "disease."

Before I take off my scientist's hat, and put on my "human" hat, I would like to say a few things about how the cancer problem appears to me, and why I think that the answers that we are all searching for are not going to miraculously appear tomorrow.

It is characteristic of primitive man to accept totally everything that he sees around him as the natural course of events, and to view anything different as a miracle. Thus, childbirth and the growth and development of the child are viewed as a natural process, while virgin birth is considered to be a miracle. Illness is also viewed as a natural process, and the recoveries from severe illness as a miracle. To the student of nature, things are often reversed. The longer that one studies life, the more miraculous the so-called natural processes seem, and the more one wonders why congenital anomalies, cancers, tumors, and disturbances of all kinds do not occur more frequently. To the naturalist, the order of things is astounding. The physicists tell us the natural tendency of things is toward disorder. In view of this, life seems even more miraculous. In order, therefore, to understand cancer it is necessary that we know a good deal about why that order exists and how it is regulated. This is not a simple problem. Nature guards her secrets well.

To the ancients, illness was illness; and you either got well or died. The growth of scientific medicine now makes it possible to say with a reasonably high degree of probability that there are very large numbers of illnesses where your chances of dying are very slim and others where the chances of your dying are great. It is little more than a generation ago that the dread disease pneumonia became curable. The suddenness with which the cure for pneumonia came led many people to believe that all diseases may fall in much the same way—including cancer. It is of course conceivable, but it does not seem to me to be very likely. We do not have instruments that enable us to peer into the future, so the understanding or cure of cancer remains, like prosperity, always just around the corner—where it will probably remain for a long time.

It is possible to find a cure for a disease without understanding the disease itself. We can "cure" headache and fever with aspirin, but we don't know how the drug acts. The cure may come before understanding, but we can't count on it. The understanding will be valuable with or without a "cure" because it will enable us to relieve a good deal of physical and emotional anguish—as understanding always does.

The understanding of cancer will not come by itself. It will take many, many, creative scientists working in a good many fields to even make a little bit of progress toward understanding cancer. It is from these people that the ultimate understanding will come, and it is very important for the public to resist the temptation to say, "We will not support you because you are not working directly on cancer." It is even more difficult for the public to avoid this attitude because the scientist's attitude is hard to swallow. It was expressed in a toast, attributed to the Royal Society in England, that says, "Here's to our research; may it never be of any use to anyone." It is important for the public to understand that this attitude is the scientist's way of retaining his objectivity, and without this device he might easily fall into the emotional traps that often catch the experimental therapist.

What has science contributed so far? I would like to mention a few things which, although they may not seem like much, have nonetheless either contributed toward the lessening of human suffering or have offered a means for preventing it in the future. The discovery of chemical carcinogens has in a large measure prevented their introduction into our foods (butter yellow, a potent liver carcinogen, was once used to color butter). The clear demonstration that cigarette smoking causes cancer opens the way to preventing an immense amount of human suffering. The discovery (by a wine chemist) that bacteria caused disease led to the development of antiseptic surgery, which makes all of the treatments of cancer possible today. The discovery of viruses has an even greater potential for the future. There is a long list of discoveries which we now pretty much take for granted that originated as a result of creative men following their curiosity—with no therapeutic aim in mind. Stop and think of the immense impact of subjects such as genetics, biochemistry, laboratory medicine, to name just a few subjects that were not even in existence a hundred years ago.

In short, there has been an immense amount of progress made toward our understanding of life in general and cancer in particular since the turn of the century. More is on its way. There are, however, some clear dangers which might considerably impede our future progress; these are discussed in Part IV. The progress will never stop because, somehow, there are people with free minds who manage to remain active despite oppressive social systems.

Optimism with regard to the outcome of current cancer research seems to be inversely proportional to the experience of the person: Those people who have had extensive experience in this field know that we have made progress. They expect further progress, but are reasonably certain that there will be no miracles and that every bit of ground will be conquered with difficulty. Novices often think that the cure is just around the corner. I think that I felt much the same way when I was younger. A good analogy can be made with the way that people approach trout fishing. A person who has never fished before who decides to start, goes to the store and purchases some tackle and some bait. He then goes to some body of water in which he has seen fish frequently caught, and fully expects to go home that evening with a mess of fish. It comes as a surprise to him that he is not nearly as successful as he expected to be. It is no accident that 10 percent of the fishermen catch 90 percent of the fish. The experienced angler is aware of the uncertainties, has a good idea of how to go about catching what kind of fish in what area. But he knows that he will periodically get skunked, there will be times when he will have to settle for one or two small ones, and that it may be a very long time before he breaks a record or catches the lunker in his favorite fishing hole. You can be pretty suspicious of the man who tells you to make sure to have the frying pan heated up by the time he gets home. There are, of course, sure ways of catching fish. One of them is to go to a trout "catchery" in which the fish are conditioned to bite at empty hooks, and another way is to buy them at the corner supermarket. There are scientists who approach science in much the same way, and they are always successful. All you have to do is pick a problem that someone else has already solved, go over it in a slightly different way, and publish your results—and if your timing is right you can become famous. I know a number of scientists who have done this, but if I mentioned names I might make enemies of a large segment of the scientific community. I probably will anyway, since some scientists are almost sure to pick up the shoe, try it on, and find that it fits.

PART III

PEOPLE AND CANCER

Why give light to a man of grief?
   Why give life to those bitter of heart,
Who long for a death that never comes

                              Job 3:20

Believe me, God neither spurns a stainless man,
   nor lends his aid to the evil.
Once again your cheeks will fill with laughter,
   from your lips will break a cry of joy.

                              Job 8:20

Is It Cancer, Doctor?

From a drop of water, a logician could infer the possibility of an Atlantic or a Niagara without having seen or heard of one or the other. So all life is a great chain, the nature of which is known whenever we are shown a single link of it. Like all other arts, the Science of Deduction and Analysis is one which can only be acquired by long and patient study, nor is life long enough to allow any mortal to attain the highest possible perfection in it.

Sherlock Holmes, in A. Conan Doyle's *A Study in Scarlet*

A portion of the tumor that the surgeon has taken out sits in a jar of formaldehyde in the pathologist's laboratory. The tumor is now about as malignant as a dill pickle. A portion of this pickled tumor will be processed, and sliced tissue paper thin. It will be stained, and then looked at through a microscope. Depending upon the appearance of this little piece of tissue, a number of inferences will be drawn in true Sherlock Holmes style. From the appearance of the tumor under the microscope, the pathologist will give it a name. The name will infer what its properties would have been had this tumor remained in the individual. It will also infer what will probably happen to the individual if some of this tumor is still left in his body. Biologists also look at living tissues, and can learn a good deal from them. What we really want to know is how the living cells behave, not how dead cells look. It is possible to infer from the appearance of the dead tissue what occurred when it was alive. Since this is technically much simpler than the use of living tissues, the use of stained dead tissue is the tool of choice of the pathologist.

The process of deducing what the tumor on the microscope slide is goes somewhat this way: The pathologist knows, to begin with, that it is a lump of a specific size in a specific area. The fact that it is a lump and that it doesn't belong there tells him immediately that it is abnormal. The next question is, What caused the lump? There are many things that can cause the appearance of a lump, such as an infection, a foreign body (a splinter or a piece of glass), or a tumor. Infection and the reaction to a foreign body result in the appearance of certain specific types of cells, and a specific pattern of distribution of the cells. After he has ruled out infection or foreign body reaction, generally the only thing left is a tumor. He then asks how much does this tissue deviate from what would normally be in this area. If the deviation is small (the cells look relatively normal in size and shape, and the pattern in which they are distributed is also normal), the tumor is usually of the benign variety. Malignant tumors often tend to have cells that look bizarre, and the ways in which they are distributed do not conform to the normal pattern for the particular tissue. For example, a malignant tumor of the breast will have mammary gland cells penetrating into muscle or connective tissues where they are not generally found; they will be in large masses, and the cells often look bizarre. They have large misshapen nuclei, and cells are large and have a lot of RNA in their cytoplasm. For every rule, however, there are lists of exceptions. With the more common tumors, pathologists have seen so many of them that they no longer have to go through the long deductive process, but can recognize them as you would recognize an old friend or enemy. Nevertheless, someone once upon a time went through the entire deductive process, drew his conclusions, and then watched the patient to see if those conclusions were correct.

Pathologists being similar to other men, the accuracy of their predictions will depend upon their experience and general judgment. There are a lot of ifs in the prognosis for an individual with cancer. If one considers the massive number of variables, the accuracy with which many of these predictions are made is almost uncanny. Yet, there are errors made by the best and wisest of these men. They are made because many of the variables are simply not known.

Let us go back to the pickled tumor. If it was a small cancer of the skin, and if it was discovered early, the individual who had it removed can go about his business with very little concern about his immediate future. If, on the other hand, it should turn out to be one of the rapidly spreading tumors of the pigment cells of the body (a melanoma—what Solzhenitsyn calls "the queen of malignant tumors"), then he had best consider the distinct possibility that his future life span may shortly be abbreviated.

The pickled piece of tumor may be one which goes by the name of Hodgkin's disease. If the tumor is of this type, then the probability of its having been removed by surgery is very slim because cells of this tumor tend to migrate out of the original tumor mass very readily. Yet, the growth characteristics of this tumor are such that it is difficult to predict if the individual having it will survive less than one year, or up to thirty years. The treatments for Hodgkin's disease are very effective, and 20 percent of treated cases (this was before the new improved x-ray treatments) will survive beyond ten years. Furthermore, there are long periods during which the patient is free of any symptoms of the disease and functions as a normal healthy individual, yet all of the aforementioned tumors, regardless of their relative lethality, go by the common name "malignant."

There are some tumors of the brain which cannot be entirely removed; the patient generally succumbing within a short period of time. These deadly tumors (craniopharyngiomas) are referred to as benign because they lack many of the characteristics of the so-called malignant tumors.

Fundamentally, a pathologist makes his judgments on the same basis on which all judgments are made—experience. Both his own and the accumulated and recorded experience of many other pathologists. With common tumors he can draw on his own experience: "I saw 100 tumors that looked like this and most patients did or did not recover." With rare tumors he has to rely on others—the authority who may have seen a large number of rare cases drawn from many other laboratories. If the pathologist cannot draw on either his own or someone else's experience, there is little basis for a rational judgment. Sometimes a reasonable guess can be made on the basis of some of the generalities that have been derived about tumors. Judgments made on this basis are highly unreliable.

The surgeon makes similar judgments based on his experience, and the appearance of the tumor at the operating table. The probability of correct judgment increases when the surgeon and pathologist pool their experience. It goes without saying that the more extensive the experience of the surgeon and the pathologist, the more reliable their judgment will be.

What is the rationale which leads people to divide tumors into malignant or benign? For the physician, there might possibly be a reason for this oversimplification. He is sometimes faced with the decision as to how to proceed in treatment; for example, whether to amputate a limb or simply to remove a tumor. To the patient, however, it may mean completely unreasonable terror.

This simple dichotomy of malignant versus benign has misled many a scientist who thinks that there is a sharp dividing line, and that the pathologist can always make the distinction.

The limit of pathology is that, at best, it can only tell you what may happen, and what the odds are. It cannot tell you what will happen. To find that out, you have to wait and see. No one has yet devised a way of looking into the future. Two people may have identical-appearing cancers of identical size and distribution. They are treated surgically by the same operation performed by the same surgeon. One dies two years later because of the cancer, and the other dies thirty years later of a heart attack. There is no way of telling what will occur before it happens—only odds can be given about what might happen. Sometimes even the longshots pay off.

The reader would do well to remember that the tumor which is removed and placed in a bottle of formaldehyde is as harmless as a dead tiger.

The word leukemia means "white blood." It is called this because, being a tumor of circulating white blood cells, the cells, following their normal predilection, circulate, resulting in large numbers of these cells in the blood. Sometimes the cells do not circulate, but remain in the organs of origin, such as the bone marrow (the tissue inside of the bones which produces most of the blood cells), or the lymph nodes, or the spleen. When it behaves in this manner, it is referred to as aleukemic leukemia (without white blood-white blood). Leukemia is the special bailiwick of the hematologist, hematology being considered a branch of internal medicine rather than pathology. He does the same thing that the pathologist does with his piece of pickled tissue. Hematologists, however, do it with a drop of blood and a drop of bone marrow. The hematologist infers from this drop of fluid what is occurring or will occur in the entire individual.

Again, as with other types of cancer, there is a wide spectrum of ways in which these blood cell tumors behave. In the case of acute leukemia, death occurs relatively soon. In the case of the chronic forms, a person may live for many years. Leukemia is an especially tragic form of cancer because, in contrast to other cancers, it has a relatively high incidence in children.

To many research biologists, leukemia is also an exciting form of cancer because a number of viruses have been identified which cause this condition in mice. This has raised some interesting speculation that if it is a manifestation of a virus infection, then perhaps a person might be immunized against leukemia virus in much the same way as he is immunized against smallpox.

To produce leukemia with a virus, it has to be introduced into the mouse at birth. It does not produce its effect until the animal becomes an adult. If the virus is given to the animal as an adult, it produces typical immunity, but no tumors. The implication of this is that when the virus is introduced into an infant, rather than causing an infection as we know it, it enters the cell and becomes a part of the genetic material (because of this, some scientists have questioned the wisdom of immunizing babies with live virus vaccines). This, in some way, results in impaired control of cell division. While a number of viruses have been isolated from cases of human leukemia, none have been shown to cause it. Obviously, no one will attempt an experiment in which a potential leukemia virus is deliberately given to a newborn child. It is a very reasonable inference that if some forms of leukemia in mice are caused by viruses, then humans also have viruses which similarly cause leukemia. It is a reasonable inference, but is by no means proved. Could a single virus be isolated from all cases, it might be more indicative. Since many viruses cause leukemia in animals, it is probable that many viruses are also involved in human leukemia. (See chapter "Yes, Virginia, Viruses Do Cause Cancer.")

The Doctor Said, "He'll Be Dead in a Year"—and He Isn't

MIRACLE, n. An act or event out of the order of nature and unaccountable, as beating a normal hand of four kings and an ace with four aces and a king.

Ambrose Bierce, *The Devil's Dictionary*

All sorts of things are attributed to treatment which have nothing whatever to do with it. Many people have had the experience of having been given an antibiotic for some disease and having the disease disappear in about three or four days. They attribute the "cure" to those antibiotics, although there is no antibiotic that I know of that does not exert some effect in the first forty-eight hours if it is going to work at all. The first clue to the working of this mysterious cure mechanism came when my wife was about to be delivered of her first child. The baby did not come quite as quickly as expected, and my wife was getting a bit anxious. The doctor prescribed some castor oil and said that, if she did not go into labor by the following morning, to take the castor oil. She went into labor at 5 A.M. and the obstetrician pointed out that, had she taken the castor oil the previous evening, the delivery would have been attributed to the treatment.

The second case in point is the case of my son's warts. He had been bothered with them for some time, and my wife consulted our pediatrician about their treatment. He gave her a prescription for some medicine which he assured her would work. The prescription worked wonders—but we never filled it. It was a week or two before she was ready to have it filled at the one and only pharmacy that made this remedy up; but by that time the warts had all disappeared.

I am now going to discuss the spontaneous cure of cancer. Spontaneous is a very fancy word which means "something that happens for which we have no explanation." But if this "cure" happens after someone has tried some worthless treatment, the patient figures that the doctor, or whoever it was, had cured him.

Occasionally some people recover from "incurable" cancer without surgical or medical intervention. This is part of the basis of the reputation of many quack cancer healers, shrines, and the power of prayer. Most of these people never had cancer at all. They either think they had cancer, or have been diagnosed as having cancer by people who were incompetent or mistaken. Of the remainder, a few represent questionable diagnosis.

There are, however, rare cases where people have been diagnosed as having cancer by the unanimous opinion of expert pathologists and have still recovered. There is no way of explaining this. *It is a fact.*

How can this occur? Perhaps part of the answer may be found in the experimental fact that we sometimes cannot distinguish changes in cell populations, which are a function of a genetic change in the cell itself, from changes which occur as a result of some change in the whole animal. If a pellet of estrogen (female sex hormone) is implanted in certain strains of guinea pigs, they develop what looks like metastatic fibrosarcoma (a rapidly spreading cancer of the connective tissue). If the pellet is removed, the tumors disappear. In some strains of rats, a similar pellet of a synthetic female sex hormone (stilbestrol) will induce the appearance of "breast cancer." When the pellet is removed, these tumors disappear. A similar phenomenon might occur very rarely in human beings. We do not know what causes these miraculous cures; we can only guess, and guesses based on very little knowledge are highly unreliable.

It is a fairly common occurence for patients to undergo what is called remission. Remission means that the symptoms, and sometimes the tumor, disappear for a period of time. This disappearance of symptoms or tumor may be of a relatively long duration (in Hodgkin's disease it can be as long as ten years) or can be relatively short. Usually remissions occur following some form of treatment, and sometimes they occur without medical intervention. In the hands of the inexperienced, a remission is sometimes taken as a cure—which it is not. In evaluating experimental treatment, the only way to tell a remission from a cure is to wait for a long enough time and see if the tumor reoccurs. If a remission follows some treatment (worthless or not), the treatment is usually considered to be successful.

Another thing worth remembering is what I have been talking about as "competing risks" in the chapter "Chemical Carcinogenesis." If a person is treated for breast cancer and dies of a heart attack two years later, the breast cancer can be considered as "cured."

When in Doubt, Cut It Out!

Removing parts of people is
The surgeon's wondrous knack.
But once the part has been took out,
It's hard to put it back.

A fairly good principle in the treatment of tumors is the surgeon's law of "When in doubt, cut it out." Many people prefer to stew and fret about little lumps before finally making the decision to see a doctor. The rationale for this seems to be that "I am afraid that it is cancer and, if it is, I don't want to know about it." The delay simply prolongs the mental agony and endangers the person's life. If the operation is not dangerous, it never hurts to remove a tumor. If it is removed, you will be relieved of future worry should it turn out, as it usually does, to be of the benign variety. Should it be malignant, then the chances of a cure are much better if it is removed early.

I am talking now about small growths on the skin or under the skin that can easily be removed with a local anesthetic. When it comes to tumors that require major surgery, that's another story. The danger of the operation has to be equated against the possibility of doing some good by it. This is a very difficult decision to make. The better the judgment and skill of the surgeon, and the judgment of the pathologist, the better the chances for the patient. Unfortunately, there is no foolproof way of determining either. (See chapter "How to Pick a Doctor," p. 142.)

What is the relationship of the size of a tumor to its curability and to its tendency to metastasize? It is surprising, in view of the importance of this question, that so little fundamental research has actually been done in this area. It makes sense to remove a tumor while it is still small because (1) the surgery is much simpler, and (2) even if the tumor has a tendency to metastasize, the probability of catching the tumor before it has actually done so is greater.

There is some fairly good empiric evidence that the smaller the tumor is when it is removed the better are the chances of survival for the patient. Survival in breast cancer treated with radical mastectomy is related to the size of the tumor when it was removed. If the tumor is less than 2 cm. (¾ of an inch) in diameter, then five-year survival is about 76 percent; if it is 2–5 cm. (¾ to 2 inches) in diameter, the five-year survival is 55 percent; and if the tumor is 5–10 cm. (2–4 inches) in diameter, then the five-year survival is about 25 percent.

If most people knew what an amazingly large percentage of cancers are completely curable by surgery (the cure rates in some forms of cancer are over 90 percent), there would be no hesitation about going to a doctor and having the operation done as soon as possible.

I would like to make it clear that I am not advocating the removal of moles, birthmarks, and other common skin lesions. We all have some of these and, if we had them all removed, not only would we be covered from head to toe with band-aids, but every surgeon and physician in the country would be kept busy removing moles. What I am referring to are the moles—or whatever you call them—that have been doing nothing for a long time which start to grow; or moles that are in areas where they are continually subject to irritation. What I should say is, If it's starting to grow, or if it is bothering you, cut it out. There is little point to "prophylactic surgery" per se. We know that we could prevent all breast cancer by removing the breasts of all women at puberty, but I don't think that anyone would advocate this as a routine procedure.

The major problem in evaluating the effect of treatment on cancer is the fact that the course of the disease is so damnably unpredictable. One woman with completely untreated breast cancer may succumb six months after diagnosis, while another may live beyond five years. In untreated breast cancer, 85 percent of the women diagnosed as having it will live for a year; 50 percent will live for two and a half years, and 20 percent will live past five years (the usual criterion for the cure of the disease). Every surgeon who has treated breast cancer knows that some of his cases succumb very quickly after surgery, while some survive for relatively long periods of time. He has no idea whether extended survival is because of his treatment, or in spite of it. The tragedy is that information on the effectiveness of surgical treatment is not that difficult to obtain; all that is necssary is that some funds be made available to the right people to do, in surgery, what is presently being done in the evaluations of the chemical treatments for cancer.

To give you some idea of what can be expected in untreated cancer, Figure 6 shows the survival curves for a number of common types of untreated cancer. This method of graphing survivors is very useful, because the slope of the line at any particular point is the death rate. The reason that we use the logarithm of the percent survival is to correct for the fact that we have a continually decreasing population. For example, if we started out with 100 people, at the end of a particular interval we would have 90, then 70, and so on. In order to have the slope of the curve equal the mortality rate, we use a logarithmic scale to correct for this decrease. The use of logarithms is not simply a gimmick, but is a valid method of correcting for the fact that the population at risk is continually decreasing.

We can view the curve as we do a sleigh riding hill, with the steepness of the slope being proportional to the speed of the sled—or the risk of dying. Take breast cancer for example: you will find that you sort of have to push your sled a bit to get started over the first year (there is not too much risk of dying in that period of time); and then it starts going down pretty

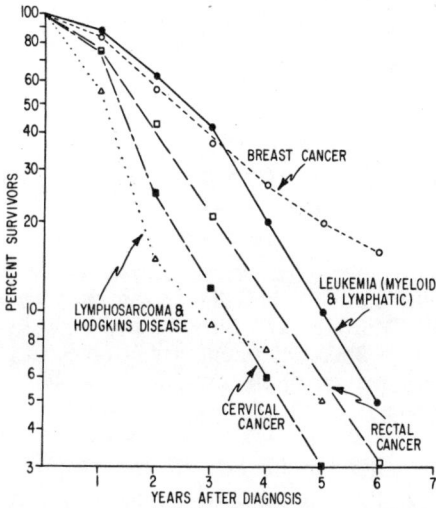

FIGURE 6

Survival of people with untreated cancer. (Data adapted from M. B. Shimkin, "Natural History of Neoplastic Disease," *The Physiopathology of Cancer*, 2nd ed., edited by F. Homburg, pp. 855–871 (New York: Harper & Row, Publishers, 1959).

fast, with the risk of dying increasing at a fairly rapid rate. By the time five years have arrived, approximately 80 percent of the untreated cases will have succumbed. The slope does not change too much even at the five-year point. If, however, you compare this curve with cases of breast cancer treated by surgery (Figure 7) you find that the slope is much more gradual, with about 60 percent of the people surviving for five years instead of the 20 percent in the untreated group. When the slope got to be about the same as the general death rate of people in the same age group that did not have breast cancer, then a person is "home free." In other words, if a woman has breast cancer and is treated, and she makes it past six or seven years, she is pretty well out of the woods. In fact, if she makes it to five years, and the doctors can detect no sign of metastasis she is also pretty well out of the woods.

So, if we wanted to find out whether a certain treatment

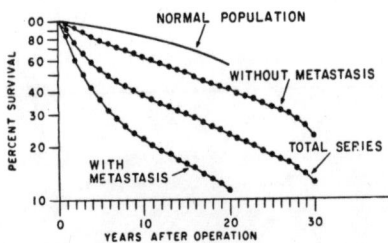

FIGURE 7

The survival of patients with *treated* breast cancer compared with the survival of the normal population in the same age group. (From J. Berkson et al., "Mortality and Survival in Surgically Treated Cancer of the Breast: A Statistical Summary of Some Experience of the Mayo Clinic." *Proceedings of the Staff Meetings of the Mayo Clinic* 32 [1957]: 647:670.)

for cancer was effective or not all that would be necessary would be to, first, draw a curve of treated cases and compare it with the curve for the untreated ones; and, second, once we have a treatment that appears to work, then we can compare the curves for individuals treated in this way with the curves for individuals treated by any new treatment. It is important to make sure that the composition of people in the groups being compared is truly comparable. To do this, the ages of the patients, the method of selection, the histologic tumor type, the stage of the development of the disease, all have to be comparable in the groups being compared. It looks complicated, but it is nowhere near as difficult and as complicated as it sounds. If an experimental treatment is used, and it is compared with a standard curve (usually the best available current treatment) and it is found that the curves overlap, it means that the addition to the treatment is ineffective. If the curve of the treated sample falls below the curve for the others, then the treatment is worse; and if the curve is above the standard curve then the treatment is better. The more times the experiment is repeated with the same results, the more believable the results become. The medical literature is full of reports where a physician tries a treatment on five or ten cases and reports superb results, which could not subsequently be obtained by others. It is sad, but true, that while the physician is the man best equipped to treat people with cancer, he is generally poorly equipped to evaluate the results of his treatment. In fact, because of built-in bias—he wants the treatment to succeed—he should leave the evaluation to unbiased statisticians. This is being done in some of the better research cancer institutes; but with their limited number of cases it will take them a lot longer to get the information needed than would a cooperative program involving many large hospitals.

I would like to anticipate my own conclusions, and point out that a cure is *not* just around the corner and we had better start perfecting the tools at hand so that, even if we can't save too many more lives, we can at least reduce some human suffering caused by ineffective treatments.

Radical Surgery

Often the less there is to justify a traditional custom the harder it is to get rid of it.

Mark Twain

The word radical has many meanings (*radix* means "root" in Latin). One of the meanings is "treatment directed to the cause" or "going to the root of a process." It also conveys the impression in cancer surgery of the cancer being a growth with many roots, and radical surgery removes those roots. The word has undergone much the same evolution in medicine as it has in politics; so while the word radical originally referred to "getting at the root" of the tumor, it now often refers to extreme surgery in which large amounts of normal tissue are removed along with the tumor—the opposite of conservative. The theoretical basis for radical surgery is that if you remove both the primary tumor and the seeds of metastasis in the adjacent lymph nodes, there should be a better chance of curing the disease.

The most frequently used radical operation is radical mastectomy: the removal of the breast and a large amount of adjacent tissue including the largest chest muscle and the lymph nodes in the arm pit (axillary lymph nodes). This eighty-year old operation is the treatment of choice for "curable" breast cancer, regardless of the type, location, stage of invasion.

Some surgeons question whether the removal of so much

"healthy tissue" is necessary to cure a cancer. There are more complications following radical mastectomy than following the simpler operations and still more complications if radiation is used with it; how much depends on the ability of the surgeon, and whether the surgery is used with radiation therapy. There is little question that the less radical the surgery, the fewer the complications that are generated by the surgery itself. If a simpler procedure worked equally well, it should be the method of choice.

Since we have little real understanding of what makes tumors grow and spread, it is necessary to evaluate treatment empirically. To do this, it is necessary to eliminate as much bias as possible from experiments. We know that no two surgeons are equally skillful, and that everyone has his own particular bias. One surgeon may believe that radical mastectomy is the only treatment, and another may believe that simple mastectomy, or simple tumor removal, will have the same results. These attitudes will not only affect the outcome of the surgery, but the emotional state of the patient. It is very easy to "prove" a theory by selecting the proper cases for each operation. Valid experiments use a group of surgeons; each one performing all of the different operations—except that the surgeon is told, by means of some predetermined system, which operation he is to perform. The results can then be analyzed by using statistical methods applicable to such "randomized" and "prospective" experiments.

In 1959 S. S. Smith and A. C. Meyer reported the survival rates of 448 patients with breast cancer that were treated by simple and radical mastectomy in Rockford, Illinois. Their data were later analyzed in 1961 by Michael Shimkin and his coworkers. Shimkin, who is both a physician and a statistician, dealt with the fact that the two sets of data would have to be comparable. If, for example, only the less severe appearing cases are subject to the simpler operation, then the data would be biased in favor of the simpler operation. They analyzed the cases by the clinical stage of the disease and found that roughly the same types of tumors were found in the groups treated with the radical operations as with the simple ones. In analyzing these data there was no evidence found that radical mastectomy resulted in better patient survival than simple mastectomy; if anything, it was the other way around. These authors concluded, conservatively, that a truly objective evaluation could now be attempted without jeopardizing the lives of any of the patients. George Crile (1964) performed a relatively uncontrolled experiment at the Cleveland Clinic. He operated on his patients with a simple mastectomy, and compared the results with those of his colleagues who used the radical procedure. He found that a larger percentage of patients treated with simple mastectomy survived longer. Following the studies of R. McWhirter (1964), D. Brinkley and J. L. Haybittle (1966) performed a well-controlled prospective experiment on the treatment of moderately advanced (Stage II) cancer of the breast. They compared, as did McWhirter, radical mastectomy with irradiation with simple mastectomy plus x-irradiation. The five-year survival was 65 percent with a simple mastectomy plus irradiation, against 52 percent with a radical. There was no question in the minds of the authors about the superiority of the simpler operation (used with irradiation). The results were so unequivocal that they discontinued the experiment and inaugurated the simpler operation as their treatment of choice "for humanitarian reasons." When I evaluated their data using an actuarial method that indicates mortality rates, it is evident that these differences are not due solely to early mortality, but are due to actually divergent death rates. In other words, the patients do better throughout the whole time period studied, with the most favorable results appearing five and six years following treatment. Despite these studies, no large objective study was undertaken in this country.

In 1970 (Fisher et al., 1970) a report was published of an analysis of the effect of radiotherapy following radical mastectomy in the treatment of breast cancer. This was a prospective study in which a valid statistical analysis could be performed and valid conclusions could be reached. Fisher and his coworkers found that the use of radiation after radical mastectomy did not improve survival. In other words, in terms of survival, radiation was of no value (it also produces complications).

Some surgeons are now doing what is known as a "modified radical mastectomy." The operation spares the pectoralis muscle and at the same time involves the removal of most of the lymph nodes. At the present time, the available evidence indicates that this procedure may be as effective as the removal of the breast, the pectoral muscles, and the lymph nodes. The data are by no means conclusive.

You may question why I present the work of a few groups of doctors weighed against the prevailing "mass of medical opinion." It is simple: these groups have cited evidence. The "mass of medical opinion" is just that—"opinion." The only studies that are relevant are those which objectively compare two procedures.

Radical mastectomy is so firmly entrenched that most surgeons would feel that they were doing a patient an injustice to perform anything but that particular operation. There is no question that it works, and that cancer has been cured by it—but so does the simpler operation.

There are some cases of breast cancer in which no treatment will work and the outcome will be fatal regardless of treatment (there is no way of identifying these). Of the remaining (potentially curable) ones, there may be a few in which the removal of tumors and lymph nodes might be more effective than simple removal of the breast. In the majority of treatable cases, the simple removal of the breast may be just as effective.

In the mouse, we know that if we take a tumor out of one part of the breast, another may crop up in another part. The same may be true of the human breast. If this is so, then the removal of the entire breast—indeed the removal of both breasts—may very well be prophylactic. I find this argument very hard to buy, because it is analogous to saying that the best prophylaxis against automobile accidents is suicide. If it could be shown that the odds of the woman developing an *untreatable* breast cancer following the surgical removal of a treatable one was very high, removal of both breasts might make sense, but there is little good evidence available at the present time. The available data indicate that the odds are in the neighborhood of 1 in 40. This could be considered a high risk in a young woman, but a low one in an old woman.

There has not, to date, been an objective test of simple tumor removal (lumpectomy), although it has been tried and reported as effective. It is not likely that there will be a decent trial until the question of radical versus simple mastectomy is unequivocally settled. At the present time, a woman with breast cancer is likely to lose her breast regardless of the size of the tumor or the type of cancer.

The radical operation currently in use was originated by Halsted in 1889 and has been gospel ever since. It does little good to point out that the available evidence shows no advantage of radical surgery over simple mastectomy. Radical mastectomy is the treatment of choice in the same way as bleeding was the treatment of choice for a wide variety of ills several centuries ago; and the same way as sweating was prescribed for fevers, gargling for sore throats, and tincture of iodine for almost everything else, forty years ago. It is the usual course of the history of medicine and science that a few individuals are far ahead of their colleagues, and that it takes at least twenty years for the rest to catch up.

Offhand, one would believe that the advent of a better treatment would be greeted by the medical profession with open arms. This is basically true about brand-new treatments such as the artificial kidney, kidney transplant, skin transplant, antibiotics, and so on. There are, however, a few innovations which the medical profession finds difficult to accept. They are the ones that require the admission of a certain amount of culpability. For a physician, who has devoted his entire life to helping people, to have to admit to himself that a treatment that he has been using has either maimed or killed some of his patients is the most difficult thing that he can possibly do. When it was discovered that radiation caused both mutation in the germ cells and leukemia, an attempt was made to persuade radiologists to protect those parts of their patients that do not have to be irradiated. A lead apron over the gonads was encouraged and as complete a lead shielding of infants as was possible. Dentists x-raying teeth could, by placing a lead apron on the laps of their patients, protect the gonads from irradiation. Some physicians and dentists finally did this in response to public pressure, saying that "If we do not do this for the patients, they will not want x-ray." Some did it in a sincere effort to protect their patients. Why this resistance? Because, in order to protect their patients, it required the admission that what they had been doing before was wrong and possibly injurious. For a physician or dentist to admit to himself that he might perhaps have caused the development of an abnormal or leukemic child is anathema. It is psychologically easier not to admit it, and to continue doing the same thing, than to admit to a lack of knowledge and change. Before it is possible to alter a fixed opinion, it is first essential to admit to the possibility that the opinion might be wrong. For a surgeon to admit to himself that a procedure which he was taught was the best possible treatment for cancer might conceivably involve the unnecessary mutilation of a patient takes a kind of courage that few people are capable of.

This indictment of the current treatment of breast cancer is all the more poignant because of one very important intangible. We have no way of knowing how many women with early breast cancer might have visited the doctors sooner had they not been afraid of losing their breast as a consequence. It is possible that, even if a simple removal of the tumor were not quite as medically effective as the removal of the entire breast, more lives might ultimately be saved by the use of the simpler operation because women would have the tumors removed earlier.

One of the most important things to consider in deciding which treatment to have for cancer is, *What are the consequences of making a wrong decision?* In the case of breast cancer, treating the cancer by removing the lump (lumpectomy) will spare the breast, and may or may not cure. If the wrong decision is made (the cancer would have been cured by removing the breast but not by removing the lump), the tumor will spread resulting in death. The equation consists of possible cure and keeping the breast against possible not cure and death. Our information at this time is that more cures will be obtained by removal of the breast. If, therefore, living is the only (or major) consideration for you, then the only reasonable procedure is to have the breast removed. If you would rather accept an added risk of dying than losing a breast, then lumpectomy is your choice. Decisions about removal of both breasts or prophylactic surgery such as the removal of the colon in chronic ulcerative colitis should consider the probability of making a wrong decision and its consequences.

What if a surgeon wants to do an operation on you that you do not wish to have done; what are your choices? The canons of medical ethics state that a physician cannot give a patient a treatment the patient doesn't want. In other words, the patient can always say "No!" Faced with this refusal, your physician can try to persuade you of the wisdom of his position —a very reasonable thing to do. He may consider things from your point of view and propose some other reasonable alternatives; or, he can say "I will not treat this condition the way you would like; you will have to go to someone else." All of these alternatives are reasonable, and allow the patient a reasonaby free choice. With the exception of abortion, and some sterilization operations, one can almost always find a physician who will administer the treatment that you consider reasonable. You must, however, be careful, because there are some physicians who will do anything for a buck. Often this is coupled with incompetence.

Signs of reasonableness are appearing among surgeons which may well have been nonexistent twenty or thirty years ago. I know a surgeon who believes that radical mastectomy is still the best treatment for breast cancer. When someone comes to him and says, "Doctor, do what you think best," this is the treatment that he administers. If, however, after carefully discussing the problem with his patient and presenting his own point of view, the woman in question wants a simpler operation, he is willing to go along with it—and he does a very competent job.

I posed a hypothetical question to another surgeon: "What

, would you do if a woman comes to you with a tumor of the breast that was less than 1 inch in size, and she stated unequivocally that she did not, under any circumstances, want her breast removed?" He said that this offered him a reasonable alternative. He would prefer the usual operating room procedure of taking a frozen section (this is a piece of tissue that is taken at the operating table and examined quickly by a pathologist), followed, if it was malignant, by a radical mastectomy. If, however, the woman refused to have her breast removed, then he said that he would remove the lump using a local anesthetic, and would send the specimen to a pathologist for examination. Should the tumor prove to be benign, that would be the end of it. On the other hand, if the pathologist declared it to be of the malignant variety, he would try to persuade the woman of the wisdom of having a radical mastectomy at that time. I told him that I was under the impression that this was not the way that it was generally done, and he replied that this was the way in which he, and the colleagues in his institution, trained surgeons. In other words, the treatment that a woman receives for breast cancer can, in a large measure, be determined by her attitude at the time that she visits a surgeon. If she is adamant about not having her breast removed, it would take a very unreasonable man to refuse her the simplest possible operation. Most patients are unwilling to make life and death decisions (or what they envision to be life and death decisions) for themselves, and prefer to have them made by others. I know that I don't feel this way, and I'm sure there must be a reader or two who thinks in much the same way that I do. I also know that my attitude would be quite different if I had small children, from what it would be if my children were all grown. I might be more willing to take a chance if there were no small children depending on me.

Flexibility is laudable, but unfortunately, it is not too common. I know an excellent surgeon who has this flexible attitude about every conceivable operation—except breast cancer.

With most forms of cancer, it is deadly to delay making a decision. Nevertheless, no matter what decision you make, you are the one who has to live with it. Get the best information that you can, weigh it against your own sense of values, and decide. The only option that you should not allow yourself is the option of doing nothing. When a woman is past the childbearing age, and someone recommends that she have her uterus removed for cancer, it is usually not as great a decision to make because she is weighing her life against the loss of an organ for which she has no further use. In a woman who intends to have children, this is a much more difficult decision to make; and with regard to losing a breast it may be more difficult. At the present time there are no conclusive answers. As with all human decisions there is no way of achieving anything approaching certainty.

We know that the probability of a cure is related to the size of the tumor when it is taken out; the larger the tumor the less the chance of the surgical cure. The chances of a cure drop about 10 percent for each increase of 1 cm. (⅜ of an inch) in tumor diameter. In view of this, you are probably better off having a lumpectomy while the tumor is less than an inch in diameter than you are having a radical mastectomy when the tumor is 2 inches or more in diameter. If the fear of losing your breast causes you to delay seeing a doctor and having surgery, find yourself a doctor that will remove the lump while it is still small and will spare your breasts—and good luck.

If you find yourself impaled on the horns of a dilemma and can't decide between radical mastectomy, simple mastectomy, or lumpectomy, *DO NOT DELAY—HAVE THE LUMP REMOVED IMMEDIATELY* and make the other decisions afterward.

Chemotherapy and Radiation Therapy

The blind artillery which cuts down its own men with the
same pleasure as it does the enemies.

Aleksandr I. Solzhenitsyn, *Cancer Ward*

What makes a cancer grow is an imbalance between M, the rate
at which cells are produced, and L, the rate at which cells are
lost. (See chapter "Anything Grows," p. 6.) In theory, treatment can be directed at either preventing or slowing down cell
division or increasing the rate of cell loss. Any treatment which
can permanently decrease the rate of cell division (without
doing the same thing to all of the other cells of the body), or
can permanently increase the rate of cell loss, would be potentially able to chemically cure a cancer. Most treatments for
cancer do not alter these rates at all. What they do is to prune
back the tumor (if you remember the diagram, what they do is
to empty the bucket). If the surgery or therapy is successful,
the entire tumor is removed so that there are no longer any
tumor cells left to divide.

The ideal therapeutic agent would act like penicillin or the
sulfonamides, and would selectively kill or inhibit the tumor
cells without simultaneously destroying the normal ones. The
major problem in finding a drug that will do this can be seen
by pointing out some of the differences between bacteria and
cancer cells. It is well established that penicillin and the sul-

fonamides kill or inhibit the vast majority of the organisms that they are supposed to attack, but not all (there are always a few left over). The genetic variability in bacteria (and tumor cells) is such that there are inevitable variants that are resistant to the drug. In the case of bacteria, the remaining organisms are taken care of by the natural body defenses. In the case of cancer cells, the cells are identical to, or sufficiently similar to, the normal cells of the animal's body so that the individual does not react against them. Any cells that are resistant to the drug and are left over will grow and start the tumor growth cycle all over again, except that this time the cells that grow are resistant to the drug that was used against them. The same principle also holds true for the use of radiation.

In theory it should be possible to prune a tumor way back with one drug; prune the remnant of the tumor with another, and so on, until—like the Cheshire Cat in Alice in Wonderland—there is nothing left but the grin, and that soon disappears. The only trouble with this approach is that while you are doing this to the tumor, you are simultaneously doing the same thing to the normal cells, so that when the tumor disappears, so does the patient—a mere detail to "Alice" fans.

As I've stated, the effect of radiation and chemicals is to destroy a large number of cells. One would ordinarily suppose that this would always be a good idea. The problem is not as simple as it seems. For example: suppose we were dealing with a tumor that had a doubling time of one week (the tumor would double its size in that time). If we could only manage to kill half of the cells, it would make a difference of one week in the life of the patient. If you could kill 99 percent or 99.99 percent, it might make a considerably greater difference in the life of the patient. If, on the other hand, we had a tumor that had a doubling time of one year and you reduced the mass of the tumor by half, it would make a difference of one year to the patient. The effect of radiation and chemotherapy is usually severe illness for a period of time. In order, therefore, to predict whether the radiation were worth using, one would have to know two things: (1) What the doubling time of the tumor is, and (2) What percentage of the cells are destroyed by the radiation. The doubling time of the tumor can be calculated by measurements of the tumor, but there is no real way of knowing what the sensitivity of the cells to radiation is. The approach used is generally empiric. There is some information about the past behavior of specific types of tumors in response to radiation or chemicals. Some types of tumors are more sensitive than others.

There is one important exception to these generalizations. The rare tumor called choriocarcinoma is a cancer usually derived from placental tissue that remained after a baby was born, or an abortion had taken place. This tissue continues to invade the uterus, and sometimes metastasizes. Since this tissue is genetically the same as the baby rather than the mother, it is "different." It therefore responds to treatment in the same way as do bacteria. The chemicals can kill it; and since it is genetically different, the individual bearing it also attacks it immunologically. This tumor can often be completely cured by chemotherapy.

A second possible exception is tumors caused by distinctive viruses. In experimental tumors in mice, when a virus causes a tumor, there is some of the individuality of the virus that is transmitted to the cell surface, such that the cells are immunologically different from the cells from which they originated. It is conceivable that this difference can be exploited, and that chemotherapy might prune back the tumor to the point where the individual's defense system can take over and destroy the rest of the cells. This may be the key to some of the apparent successes in the chemical treatment of acute leukemia, and a tumor called Burkitt's lymphoma.

Very little has been tried in the way of reeducating cancer cells back to a normal state. To do this successfully, one would have to understand the normal physiology of the cell, and what went wrong with it. Until we reach this point, we will have to resort to the usual primitive approach to an enemy—kill; unfortunately, in attacking the enemy, one also attacks the patient.

One thing becomes apparent from reading the literature,

and talking to a variety of physicians: The chemical treatment of cancer is sufficiently complex and new that it should no more be trusted to the general medical practitioner than should heart surgery. There are relatively few physicians who have the know-how to treat cancer with chemicals, and these are almost exclusively located in either major cancer or medical centers. There is little question that an individual with a curable type of tumor would do better at one of these centers. With tumors that can only be palliated, one must weigh the relative advantages of going to a treatment center against the personal advantages of staying home. It is always a good idea for a patient with cancer to go to one of these centers to find out what they have to offer. It may be very little, or it may be a great deal. Most practitioners aren't too well informed on what is available.

The therapeutic use of x-ray works on the principle that if you can't cut it out, kill it. Many radiotherapists, having an evangelistic streak, feel that it's better to kill it where it sets rather than take it out and then kill it. A knife, however, is much more selective than a radiation beam with regard to what it kills.

I asked a surgeon whose judgment I respected how he would have his wife treated for cancer of the uterine cervix. He said that surgery would be his choice if he knew a first-rate surgeon in a good modern hospital. If there was any question, he would prefer taking his chances with radiation therapy— even with a mediocre radiotherapist. I asked the same question of a radiologist, and he said that he'd prefer a mediocre surgeon to a mediocre radiotherapist.

The legitimate uses of radiation are almost exclusively on tumors that cannot be reached surgically. Radiation is effective on tumors of cells of the defense system (the tumor called Hodgkin's disease) and with incurable tumors which can be reduced in size with radiation. There is no question but that radiation works, and that it has prolonged the lives of some people with cancer. It reminds me of the story of the man who was playing roulette and was asked by a friend if he didn't know that the roulette wheel was rigged. He replied, "Of course

I know the game is fixed." "Then why do you play it?" asked his friend. And his reply was, "Because it is the only wheel in town!"

Since x-rays also produce cancer, it's not a good idea to use them if there is another equally effective way of treatment (provided that the risks are comparable). This is particularly true with regard to its use on children and young adults.

The Scientist and the Therapist

To the ancient aphorism, first do no harm, should be added
a modern extension: compassion without competence is crap.

Michael B. Shimkin, Report from Laputa,
"Some Polemics on Medical Mythology,"
Archives of Environmental Health, 22:151–153 (1971).

The cancer research scientist is a chronic doubter—he is never
sure what he is looking for, nor what he wants to find. The
experimental cancer therapist knows what he is looking for
and what he wants to find—but he needs the scientist to tell
him where to look. The scientist is apt to be a doubter, the
therapist a true believer. The scientist is suspicious, even
angry, with the therapists's evangelism, and the therapist is
impatient with the scientist's equivocation and criticism. The
rare individual who does both leads a schizophrenic existence.
Usually, he forsakes one calling for the other, or goes into
administration (and often very effectively, since he understands the problems of both groups).

The objective critic of the experimental therapist can
sometimes be impaled on the horns of a dilemma by an unscrupulous experimental therapist.

- If the critic asks for adequately controlled experiments,
he is reminded that the therapist is a physician, i.e., he cannot
withhold a possible cure.

- If the critic points to the basic doctrine of the humane
physician—above all, do no harm (*primum non nocere*)—he

is informed that science takes precedence over the physician's art.

• When the contradictions in the above arguments are presented, the critic is then reprimanded for criticizing someone who is "at least *trying* to do something."

Experiments that harm patients deserve to be criticized regardless of the motivation. Most practitioners are humane physicians who try; and if they fail to produce a cure or alleviate symptoms, they comfort relatives, relieve suffering, and allow their patients to die with dignity. There are also sadists and cancer quacks with and without M.D. degrees, both in and out of respectable institutions, who deserve to be tarred and feathered.

Treatments, for good or evil, are much like laws—they are easy to institute and hard to repeal. Current medical history is full of treatments that hurt and kill people. In my lifetime, I have seen the following:

1. X-ray given to shrink the thymus gland of infants. Results: did the children no good and subsequently caused leukemia and cancer of the thyroid in some.

2. X-ray for a whole variety of lesions, including warts (which can be wished away) and ankylosing spondylitis (a disease of the spine). Results: the lesions disappeared and the leukemia rate increased.

3. High oxygen to premature infants. Results: blindness in some.

4. Removal of the tonsils. Results: in some cases, very helpful, but in most cases, unnecessary (even in preantibiotic days). Some operative deaths (percentagewise low; in actual numbers of deaths, considerable).

5. Antibiotics for colds. Results: does no good for colds. Can cause sickness and death in allergic patients; destroys normal bacteria needed for resistance to other diseases.

6. Antibiotics for virus infection. Results: in most cases either worthless or potentially harmful.

7. Injection of plastics for cosmetic reasons. Results: experimental evidence indicates that the probable long-term result will be cancer in those treated.

8. Thalidomide as a tranquilizer (not many in the U.S.). Result: deformed children when used in early pregnancy.

9. Stilbestrol in early pregnancy. Result: cancer of the vagina in female children of women so treated (see chapter "Chemical Carcinogenesis.")

These are easy to document. There is a long list of probably harmful treatments and a longer list of possibles.

There is sometimes a conflict between what is preferable in the treatment of patients and what is needed to be scientific. There may be times when the appropriate application of the scientific method, to the detriment of the patient, may prove to be beneficial to a much larger number of people. I am, therefore, willing to accept an institution that practices good medicine and poor science, or one that practices poor medicine and good science. I have no patience with one that practices neither good medicine nor good science.

A physician friend of mine says that it would be better to concentrate my criticism on the out-and-out cancer quack, rather than the medical profession. I disagree: The con man is not going to improve as a consequence of public pressure —some members of the medical profession might. It is because the physician is conscientious and trying to do the best for his patient that improvement is possible. The only thing that can be done in this book about the cancer quack is to warn the public—and this has already been done many times.

Almost all judgments in clinical medicine are tentative and almost all treatments are experimental. That is a pretty dogmatic statement—let me explain:

The reason that I say that most judgments are tentative, is because it is still impossible to predict the future. The perceptive physician is aware of this, and continually follows his patient through the course of treatment, changing it when necessary. It is reasonably well established that penicillin is one of the best treatments for infection. However, in administering the treatment, the physician may find out that the organism that he is trying to kill appears to be resistant to the drug, or the patient may be allergic to penicillin, making the drug potentially lethal. The perceptive physician immediately changes his treatment to another antibiotic. The one who follows scriptures will continue the treatment, endangering the life of the patient.

To say that all treatment is experimental is also a valid judgment, in the same way that all automobiles are experimental, all airplanes are experimental. Unfortunately, in the process of trying to please both himself and his client, the physician may (as General Motors did with automobiles) provide a product that is far from the best. It is also far from the worst. This point was brought home to me in a discussion with a gynecologic surgeon who believes that he is able to separate two different types of cancer of the uterus; one being 100 percent lethal, and the other relatively susceptible to treatment. He is trying radical surgery in an attempt to cure the lethal type. I questioned him about the untreated controls in his experiments and he said "I don't need any: this disease is 100 percent fatal, and if I save just one patient, we will have accomplished something." This made sense to me. His procedure is what we refer to, in the laboratory, as a "pilot" experiment which is the type of experiment that you perform when you are looking for promising leads. His answer to my next question was disconcerting. I asked him, "Suppose that out of ten patients, two get well—what are you going to do then?" His reply was, "This will become our method of treatment." At this point he and I intellectually parted company. I believe that once an experimental therapist has a procedure that works he should not rest on his laurels. The next step should be to refine the procedure to minimize the risk of injury to the patient. This would consist of a series of controlled experiments in which one group of patients received the new operation, while another group had a similar operation with some of the undesirable parts of it left out. These experiments should be continued until the best possible treatment was found—one that is lifesaving and has as few undesirable side effects as possible.

The question in my mind is not whether physicians should experiment on their patients—they do, they have to, and they will continue to do so. I would like the experiments to be well controlled so that the physicians of the future will have better and more reliable treatments than did their predecessors. Most of the experimental therapy performed today is very poorly controlled. Perhaps this is because the traditions of scientific method are new to medicine. The tradition in the healing arts consists of a belief in the dicta of "authorities." The scientific tradition, in contrast, is one of skepticism and the constant questioning of authority. Medicine (especially academic medicine) has a mixture of scientists, who often are the "authorities" and practitioners, who are, with rare and wonderful exceptions, true believers. Sometimes the scientists abandon the scientific tradition and become dogmatic authorities. There is usually a running battle in medical schools between the scientists and the practitioners, and there is nothing "scientific" about the way that it is fought. The ideal medical school professor who can be a critical scientist and a humane practitioner is rare—and one who can also teach is still rarer.

I don't know what motivates a physician to specialize in cancer therapy and I am not sure that I want to know. In the tradition in which I was raised, the noblest thing that a human being can aspire to is to help the hopeless. I do not understand how a person can do this because, even with the outer atmosphere of cheerfulness and hope, it must be a veritable internal hell for the man who has to do it. Every physician is grateful to the man who lifts the awesome burden of the incurable cancer patient from his shoulders. It must also be said that there are also therapists who thrive on human misery, whom the world would be better off without. Despite my admiration for the conscientious therapist, I cannot share his enthusiasm.

Victories of cancer therapists are small, and they come hard. The obstetrician has the joy of bringing new life into the world; the surgeon who takes out an appendix or removes a tumor successfully has the satisfaction of knowing that his patients get well. The cancer therapist, in contrast, spends most of his time giving people a little bit of added life, or making people more comfortable. He knows that most of his patients will die in a relatively short time.

These are dedicated men, driven by some inner need to

serve the hopeless. Most of them work in the tradition of Father Damien. It is these people who are dedicated to helping the hopeless who make this world a more beautiful place to live in. Yet, as is often the case, highly dedicated people can be blind to the objective truths about what they are doing.

To give a person a year or two more of life is usually a desirable thing. It is desirable if that year or two of life is relatively pain-free and the person so blessed is allowed to lead a relatively normal life. To literally bring someone back from the grave, only to have him die in pain three months later, is not only not a service, but is unnecessarily cruel. Treatment with large doses of x-ray makes patients very ill for a period of time, as do some of the chemicals used in chemotherapy. The skillful therapist is often able to make the distinction between conditions where his treatment can do some good, and those where it probably cannot. To suggest to a patient, who cannot be helped, that he not be treated might be the kind thing to do. It is, unfortunately, the rare therapist who will not treat a patient, and the patient is subjected to unnecessary discomfort. Part of the reason for his treating the patient is his enthusiasm, and part is the insistence of some patients and their relatives that the doctor "do something."

A dogma that has permeated medical practice for as long as it existed is that *anything that a physician does is better than doing nothing.* It is extremely difficult for someone who has devoted his life to helping people to admit to himself—much less to the world—that his patients might have been better off if he had never seen them. Some of the more cynical members of the thinking public have made this evident. Mark Twain's remark, "He has been a doctor a year now and has had two patients—no, three, I think—yes, it was three; I attended their funerals," testifies to this skepticism. It was well-known by the public that the great general hospital in Vienna in the first half of the seventeenth century had an extremely high mortality in pregnant women. This was due to a condition known as puerperal fever. It was Ignaz Semmelweis who showed that the infective material that caused this disease was conveyed by the hands of the doctors and medical students from the autopsy room to the expectant mother. He was virtually laughed out of the profession, and ended his days in a lunatic asylum. Perhaps it takes a madman to keep "sane people" from doing harm. A more recent example illustrates that the attitudes in medicine are slow to change. H. J. Muller discovered that x-rays produce genetic changes (mutations) in 1927. He received the Nobel Prize for this work in 1946. By that time it was also well established that x-rays could induce leukemia in mice, and that the leukemia incidence was considerably higher in radiologists than in other medical practitioners and the population at large. This had the effect of inducing radiologists to wear lead aprons when performing fluoroscopy, but had little effect on how they treated their patients. A concerted campaign was started approximately twenty years ago by a number of people in fundamental biology and radiology to induce people using x-rays to reduce the exposure to themselves and their patients. It met with unbelievable resistance and hostility. It is not possible to equate the number of people who have been sent to their death because of the use of medical x-ray against the number of people whose lives have been saved by the same tool. There is no way of estimating either.

> The blindness of the fanatic is a source of strength (he sees no obstacles) but it is the cause of intellectual sterility and emotional monotony.
>
> Eric Hoffer, *The True Believer*

Leukemia in Children

I too could talk like you,
    were your soul in the plight of mine.

                    Job 16:4

But have I the strength to go on waiting?
What use is life to me, when doomed to
    certain death?

                    Job 6:11

The considerations that apply to the treatment of cancer in adults are not quite the same as those in children. Children are not just small adults; there are many qualitative differences that justify considering them separately. Children have a different time scale—what would be a few days in bed for an adult is an eternity for a child. Since they do not have enough information to be able to make rational decisions for themselves, decisions are made for them by their parents and physicians. An adult cancer patient at age 75 may say, "I have lived my life and my time has come, and I intend to go out gracefully"; the child can neither say nor think this; by all standards, his life should just be beginning. No one can view the passing of a child with equanimity, as we sometimes can the passing of an old adult.

I talked to a hematologist with long and extensive experience in the treatment of leukemia in children. He told me that in all of his years of practice, no one has ever refused treatment for a child—even in the days when the treatment was almost totally ineffective. I have personally seen the parents of children with leukemia fleeced of every bit of savings that they had, by an unscrupulous cancer quack (this one was an M.D.) who injected their children with extracts of pineal gland that were so alkaline as to constitute the injection of a lye solution. The parade of parents with ill children to shrines in the hopes of miraculous cures is a pathetic spectacle.

If I were writing this chapter thirty years ago, I think that I could have presented a very powerful argument for parents of children with leukemia to say to their doctor, "I want no treatment for my child except that which might make him more comfortable." I can't say that now, because there is little question that chemical treatments for acute leukemia and for Burkitt's lymphoma can be effective. Many children's lives have been extended to over five years after the start of treatment. For the majority who do not make it, it was a valiant, but worthless effort—while for the few who do make it, it is the mixed blessing of life with the sword of Damocles hanging by a hair over their heads. I have no answers. I rejoice in the victories! I also know that there is very little in this world that is all good—and the announcement of a number of children who are still free of leukemia five years after having been treated, while a wonderful thing to those who are cured, cannot help but make the disappointment greater for the parents of the thousands of children who will be deprived of the benefits of living by leukemia, in spite of everything that their doctors can do. I cannot say, as has been implied many times in the press, "Rejoice, parents of leukemic children—the cure has come!"

My experience with the experimental chemotherapy of leukemia is limited to what I have seen and heard. I have not had a child with leukemia, nor have I ever been involved in treatment. I recently heard a talk by a well-known experimental therapist from Europe who described what he was doing in an attempt to "cure" leukemic children. I found it frightening. Based on experiments which, from a scientist's point of view, are of questionable value, he has injected truly therapeutic drugs into children with leukemia and also injected cells which not only attack the tumor cells, but the normal cells of the patient. The tumors occasionally disappear, but the patients die of the effects of the treatment. His apparent lack of sensitivity to the feeling of his patients was obvious in the way that he talked, and in the material that he presented.

Fortunately, I did not stop there, but talked to people in hospitals in this country. I found that, contrary to my expectations, the welfare of the patient is placed first—and only if his welfare is not jeopardized are experimental treatments used. I was impressed with the dedication and the fundamental kindness of the people involved in treating leukemia—and the fact that most of the treatments are performed on an outpatient basis, with the children being able to lead relatively normal lives during the periods when their disease is kept in check with chemicals. I could find no fault with this approach to the problem of treating leukemia in children, and the argument about the conflict between patient care and scientific method (lack of untreated controls) is one which is extremely difficult to resolve. I would not wish it resolved at the expense of the children.

What are the odds of survival in children (under 20 years of age) who develop *acute* lymphocytic leukemia? How long can we expect these children to survive, given the best treatment possible? (At the present time, it's largely the chemical treatment procedure that was started in 1966.) Survival has continually increased since 1960, and a comparison of the odds would look something like this:

The chance of a child surviving twelve months after the diagnosis has been made was such that 40 out of 100 would have done so before 1960. From 1966 on, one could expect 80 out of 100 to live for over a year.

Only 6 of 100 children would have survived to two years before 1960, and now 55 out of 100 would go that long.

I have been informed that there are more than 160 people who have had acute leukemia and have survived for over five years. I don't know what the odds are, because I don't know the size of the sample. It is a considerable number and, for the first time in history, some guarded optimism is justifiable.

With regard to the other forms of leukemia (acute myelocytic leukemia and the chronic leukemia) the effect of treatment on the outcome of the disease has been negligible. If a person is diagnosed as having acute myelocytic leukemia, one out of five people will make it to 12 months, about one out of ten to 24 months, and one out of twenty to 36 months.

The real tragedy is that the ill child is a "sure thing" for the con man. If an unscrupulous operator wishes to extract money from people, the foolproof way is to tell him that his money might help a sick or dying child. Fortunately, these unscrupulous con men are rare, but one such con man is one too many.

Stories often appear in the newspapers which tout a "new cure for leukemia." These stories invariably appear just before some organization is about to start a campaign for funds. The stories are a gold mine to the organization. The amount of suffering that these stories cause to the families of children with leukemia is immeasurable. Every time that such a story appears, doctors are deluged with phone calls and letters wanting to know about the "new cure." The heartbreak when these people are told that "it is nothing new" or "it really hasn't been tested" or "that is the treatment that your child is getting" is hard to estimate. It is considerable, totally unnecessary, and brutal. The fact that this act is done by people who are apparently unaware of the consequences does not excuse it. Newspapers and magazines could perform an act of human kindness by refusing to print press releases which contain reports of "cures" and "breakthroughs" unless they have been independently checked for authenticity. At the present rate, this would mean only one such report every five years, not several each year.

To Treat or Not to Treat

"Kostoglotov! Twelve sessions of x-rays have turned you from a corpse into a living human being. How dare you attack your treatment? You complain that they gave you no treatment in the camp or in exile, that they neglected you, and in the same breath you grumble because people are treating you and taking trouble over you. Where's the logic in that?"

"Obviously there's no logic." Kostoglotov shook his shaggy black mane. "But maybe there needn't be any, Ludmila Afanasyevna. After all, man is a complicated being, why should he be explainable by logic? Or for that matter by economics? Or physiology? Yes, I did come to you as a corpse, and I begged you take me in, and I lay on the floor by the staircase. And therefore you make the logical deduction that I came to you to be saved at any price! But I don't want to be saved at any price! There isn't anything in the world for which I'd agree to pay any price!"

Alexandr I. Solzhenitsyn, *Cancer Ward*

There are two ideas about what the role of the physician is: One holds that the role of the physician is to preserve life; the second, which I consider to be more rational, is that the proper role of the physician is to alleviate suffering. My reason for preferring the second is that we all die and there may well be things that are worse than death. The thought that keeps people alive in the middle of extreme physical pain or mental anguish is that at sometime in the future, things will be better. If a person were sure that he would spend the next year in extreme physical pain, ending in his death, it might be rational to consider suicide. Many older people have decided to forego treatment when properly informed about the probability of surviving, for how long and in what condition.

There is an aphorism in the medical profession that says that "any physician knows when to treat; the good physician knows when *not* to treat".

The final decision as to whether a patient receives treatment is best left to the patient. Someone with cancer should have the option of saying "I will take the treatments," or "I will let nature take its course." In many cases, however, the choice is really made for the patient; because, the moment the physician says "you have a chance of being cured" the patient thinks "I can take a good deal of suffering, if it means that I can live for a long time." The question of the morality of telling a patient that he has a chance of being cured depends on what the chances really are. If the odds are one in ten, then it is clearly worth taking a chance—but what if the odds are one in 100, one in 1,000, or one in 10,000; or what if the odds are about the same as that of a miraculous spontaneous recovery. At what point should a physician hold out hope of a cure? And at what point should he say "My treatment is practically worthless, but miracles do happen and you might get well"?

If you or your child is the cancer patient that the surgeons have declared untreatable, it's up to you to make the decision about further treatment. It is not necessary to feel guilty about letting nature take its course. Some very knowledgeable physicians have made just such choices about their own lives. It's your life—the choice is up to you. Insist on knowing the odds of the treatment being effective. Some people don't figure that long shots are worth it, if you calculate the cost in prolonged suffering against the merit of a quick death. It takes the ultimate in maturity to meet death without struggling. It does little good, as Dylan Thomas said, to "rage against the dying of the light." While I understand the fighters (die with your boots on), my admiration goes out to those who accept the end with serenity. I doubt that the fighters live longer or happier than the resigned—it might even be the reverse.

The therapist's values of "life at all costs" should not be the determining factor. Whether or not we wish to admit it, there are things that are worse than dying. Prolonged and painful illness exerts a profound effect on the patient and on those who love him.

Every time that experimental medicine has a success it makes the front pages: the first successful kidney transplant, the first successful heart transplant, the first few children with acute leukemia that survived beyond the expected period, and so on. This has led the general public to expect miracles as a matter of course. They do not take into account the many people who have been treated in the same way and have died— sometimes more painfully than they otherwise would have. A surgeon who has been doing kidney transplants for the past eight or ten years suggested to me that he was beginning to have his doubts about the value of what he was doing. Not that the transplants don't work, nor that he has not prolonged the lives of many people—he has. Because of his efforts, a number of people who ordinarily would have died at young ages have been living for at least five or more years. He told me that if his own kidneys failed he's not sure that he would undergo the treatment. His reason for this is the inspiring example of the few patients he has had who have refused treatment and have peacefully gone to their death. For a man who has devoted his whole life to "fighting death" to admire people who allow themselves to die is a rare and fascinating phenomenon. Young physicians almost always feel that death is the worst of all possible events. When they get older, and wiser, they sometimes come to the realization that death is not the worst thing in the world. Young physicians will often fight for days and weeks and months, to preserve the last remaining spark of life in a dying human being. Older physicians come to realize that everyone dies, and that death may well be preferable to some of the alternatives.

Several years ago I had a badly shattered leg. I was in constant pain for five months and managed to get my sleep in two- or three-hour spurts. When the sleeping pills and pain killers wore off, I was caught in the dilemma of remaining awake and in pain, or being drugged and not in pain. Most of the time I choose the first alternative, because I like to feel alive—even though at that time I was more or less faking it. What kept me going was the assurance that the leg would heal and the pain would eventually cease, which it did. There were moments when I wished that I could die for a little while. I think that if I believed that the rest of my life would be like those few months, I might very well have considered ending it all. It is a tautology to say that pain is painful—but it's true, and there is nothing quite as bad as hurting badly.

I have seen things which I consider to be worse than dying. I have seen people in unremitting pain who had no possibility of recovery; I have seen people whose brains were destroyed, who are not even able to keep themselves clean, feed themselves, or have any awareness of who they are.

While working on this book, I went to a chemotherapist to check out some information. He took me by the hand (like a child does who has just done something that he considers praiseworthy) and said, "Come, this is something that you must see!" In the examining room was a woman in her sixties. All of her hair was gone; her equilibrium was disturbed, and she was very unhappy—but in a dull way. He said, "She has lung cancer. You should have seen her a month ago. She was in coma and barely alive—look at her now." When we left the room, I asked him "How much time does she have?" He replied, "If we're lucky, maybe six months." I asked myself "How is she going to die?" "What will the rest of her life be like?" She had had a metastasis to the brain, and a brain tumor is usually a fairly painless way to go. Before the therapist treated her, she was in a coma, and it would have been a short time before she succumbed. He had brought her back to life. How is she going to die now? How much pain will she suffer? How much is she suffering now? I know of a famous pathologist who found that he had cancer of the colon. He refused any treatment and allowed nature to take its course. A surgeon once told me that he doesn't even send his patients to the chemotherapists or radiation therapists unless there is a chance that they can do something substantial; not just prolong life for a few months.

The other side of the coin is that I have a dear friend who

has incurable breast cancer. After surgery, she developed a metastasis to the brain which she had treated with radiation. The doctors thought that she had a maximum of six months. Eight months after the treatment, she tells me that she is rebuilding a cottage, putting on some weight, and feeling fine. I am glad that she had the treatment and is still alive, as are her husband and children. She is happy with her decision.

Bromides such as "always treat" or "always let them die peacefully" are not the answer. Each person should be allowed to decide for himself. It is also advisable to make the decision before being incapacitated because, once in a coma, the decision, by default, goes to someone else.

Go to a Cancer Quack—It's Your Life

How cheerfully he seems to grin,
How neatly spread his claws,
And welcomes little fishes in,
With gently smiling jaws!

Lewis Carroll,
Alice's Adventures in Wonderland

Despite the warnings of the American Cancer Society and others about the cancer quack, people pour an inestimable number of dollars into the pockets of professional and amateur con men. There is not much that you can do if somebody is willing to first buy the Brooklyn Bridge, and then jump off of it.

If, after you have gone to a reliable medical center and been told that you have incurable cancer, you then decide to take advantage of herb tea, massages, chicken soup, Q-rays, Krebiozen, and a wide variety of other totally worthless treatments, that's fine. But before you do this, make sure (1) that you have cancer, and (2) that there isn't a real cure or effective treatment for the type of cancer that you have. Most cancers are curable by surgery, and a few others by chemotherapy or radiation. Even some incurable types can be reduced in size for periods of time.

Not all quacks are blatantly dishonest—some really believe that their treatments work. There are also scientists or physicians who suddenly decide that they have found the secret to eternal life and wish to share it with mankind.

Before you go to someone who promises a cure for cancer, consider what kind of human being would experiment on people without really knowing what he is doing. What would you think if someone was lying with a broken leg, and a man who knew nothing about first aid pushed a doctor aside, saying, "Let me do it; I have the answer." There are many maniacs who feel that they have the answer to disease, old age, and so on. Their personal histories are often characteristic; a life of frustrations, unrealized ambitions, and a need—a crying need—for recognition. One cancer quack who is fairly famous in Europe was a member of the Nazi party for four years. He jumped from one thing to another, and finally ended up founding his own cancer hospital in which his own cancer treatment is used on patients, with little demonstrable effect other than fattening the purse of the man who founded the clinic.

There is always some "scientific" theory behind the treatment that every quack uses, and the controlled studies needed to prove it are always somewhere in the future—"when the money becomes available." Other doctors are always "attacking their work" and "demanding the impossible." There are always testimonials from "cured" patients, and from some "authority." A person who puts himself in the hands of one of these psychopaths doesn't know whether he will do nothing or help him to die sooner.

Every great scientist and every discovery was subject to intensive criticism by the establishment. This is, of course, true. Louis Pasteur was called a quack, as were others. It is true that new discoveries are usually treated with skepticism by science. This is as it should be, since most of these so-called discoveries will turn out to be of no value whatever. The discoveries that are valid will eventually be recognized; if not today, then within the next twenty years.

As you have no doubt gathered, I am not particularly fond of the way in which either the medical or scientific establishment operates. It is important, however, to point out that the major opposition to The Establishment does not come from outside the professions, but from within them. The problems are so complex that it takes a lifetime of experience to be able to provide intelligent opposition. The people working toward reform are themselves physicians and scientists. This is the way that it has to be. Individuals who set up their operation outside the purview of the medical or scientific establishment are invariably quacks. The mavericks who make the discoveries are themselves a part of the medical or scientific establishment. They are constantly fighting its orthodoxy, but are nevertheless part of the family. The quack, on the other hand, generally sets up his own establishment somewhere on the outside, where he is free of criticism and free to do whatever he wants to do, to anyone who will let him do it.

It is also worth remembering that the scientist or physician who finds an effective treatment for any kind of cancer profits immensely by it. He is rewarded in prestige, and ultimately financially. If his treatment is effective, he may receive the ultimate in scientific rewards. The rewards will not come until his treatment has been rigorously tested. The sooner it is tested, the sooner the rewards will be his. If he thinks that he has something, he will stop at nothing to get those critical tests performed.

Great discoveries are published somewhere in the scientific literature. They are not only subject to criticism, but are subject to critical testing. There are no excuses made—the tests are performed, and if the scientist who made the discovery turns out to be right, he is acclaimed. If he is wrong, his work is buried. In legitimate science, there is never any profit in delaying a critical test of his discoveries. In the case of the cancer quack, if the discoveries are untested, he stands to profit indefinitely from the gullibility of the people that come for his treatment. If someone is treating people without these critical tests, watch out. He is either a madman, a con man, or a fool.

There are scientists and physicians in cancer centers all over the world who are eager to test any promising lead. There are no secret cancer clinics anywhere that have anything to offer that is not already available at most cancer centers. There are no secret cures that work, there is no fountain of youth, and there is no philosopher stone that will turn lead into gold— Yes, Virginia, there is *no* Santa Claus.

The harm that the cancer quack does is indirect, in that he keeps people from receiving competent diagnosis and treatment which might cure whatever they have while it's still curable. Maybe I'm being too harsh on the cancer quack; he exists by grace of the stupidity of the people who go to see him. It takes two to play any game, and if a person wants to commit suicide, why blame the one who hands him the gun? It is strange that people who will have their car serviced by the best mechanic that money can buy will take their bodies to someone who knows and understands nothing.

How to Pick a Doctor

> I prefer my physicians to be older men with slightly jaundiced eyes. The enthusiasm of youth frightens me; and fanatical devotion to "saving lives" terrifies me.

As long as I'm giving advice about human cancer, I might as well go the whole hog and give the public the secret that the medical profession guards zealously. Many people have found this secret on their own; but some extremely intelligent people still believe that the best way to find a good doctor is to call the County Medical Society—which it isn't.

A recommendation from a number of people who have been treated successfully can often help, but is not the most reliable method in the world. Many years ago, I was bothered by hemorrhoids, which I anticipated having to have treated surgically. I inquired of people with similar complaints, and they unanimously referred me to a well-known local proctologist. Their recommendations were all the same, "He is a wonderful doctor, and does great work. I had to be reoperated twice, however." The recommendation was always glowing and the results of the surgery were always wanting. I ended up being reamed by a competent general surgeon who didn't like doing hemorrhoidectomies. I haven't been troubled with the problem since.

First of all, let us assume that your physician, no matter how competent or incompetent he is, still knows more about what is available medically than you do. The same holds true of senior residents in large hospitals.

How do you get an honest physician to give you an honest answer? If you ask the question, "Whom would you recommend to do a ......ectomy on my aging father?" the answer will usually be a local physician who refers patients to him and with whom he plays golf. This may be a perfectly reliable recommendation, since he is not likely—being an honest man—to recommend someone who is totally incompetent. On the other hand, there are varying degrees of competence (or incompetence, Dr. Peter). A better way of asking the question (which puts the doctor in a spot, since he either gives you an honest answer or has to live with his conscience for a less than honest one) is, "If *your* father needed a ......ectomy, to whom would you send him?" This is more likely to get you the doctor you are looking for—the most competent man in the area. If you happen to be living in a small town and don't have a physician you trust, a good bet is to corner the chief resident in the local large city hospital. He is forbidden, by professional ethics, to refer you to anyone; but if you make it clear that you're not asking for a referral, but simply asking an academic question such as "Who would *you* go to if you needed a ......ectomy?" you may be able to get an informative answer. Any of these methods is better than using the yellow pages.

It is now dogma that a person should see his doctor once a year and receive a physical examination. Obviously, walking up to him and saying "Hello doctor" and him answering you does not constitute an examination. There are also examinations that would take the examining physician many hours, and would involve hundreds of dollars worth of x-ray and laboratory work. If a person feels that he is in good health and has no outstanding complaints, there seems little point to going to any massive expense. There are, however, a few things in a physical examination that are simple and relatively harmless; and if something is found it might save the patient's life. Much of the credit for the reduction in death from cancer of the uterine cervix can be attributed to the use of the so-called Pap smear which can detect cancerous and precancerous conditions at times when they are easily treatable. Men and women (particularly those over forty years of age) should have a finger examination of the rectum. The finger can detect half of all tumors of the large intestine. It can also detect tumors or abnormalities of the prostate gland in the male. Many physicians prefer to use a sigmoidoscope, which is an instrument that enables the physician to visually examine the rectum. It can detect two-thirds of all tumors of the large intestine. With cancer of the bowel, the earlier that it is discovered the better the patient's chances; and it goes without saying that if they are discovered before there is any discomfort it's even better. If, in the course of the routine examination, a physician does not do a Pap smear and examination of the breast on a woman, and a rectal examination of some kind on people of both sexes, the patient is not getting much of a physical. He is probably wasting both his and his doctor's time.

Beware of physicians who promise a cancer cure. They are either trying to con you, or conning themselves. In either case, the results can be disastrous. The honest professional can give you some estimate of the odds, but that is the best he can do. In some kinds of cancer, such as early basal cell carcinomas of the skin, the odds are very high (it almost approaches certainty of a cure with tumors of less than a half an inch in diameter; the smaller the tumor the better the prognosis). With a larger tumor, your physician has no way of giving that much assurance.

Given accurate information, people are generally able to make rational decisions. Unfortunately, accurate information with regard to cancer is hard to obtain. We usually have to settle for the best "educated guesses" that are available. It is a good idea, therefore, to check out information that involves life and death decisions, before acting on it. This can often be done by obtaining a second opinion. Competent physicians encourage this. They encourage it because they are aware of their own fallibility, and would prefer to share the responsibility for a potential wrong decision. One of the best reasons for seeking a second opinion is if your physician objects to it. If he objects, make sure that the second opinion comes from someone who is not associated with your doctor.

Prevention Is Better

Cancer is not like love—It is much better to never have had any.

If we are worried about cancer, and consider it detrimental, then the single most important activity that people can engage in is its prevention. This is particularly true of the types of cancers that are highly lethal, such as leukemia and lung cancer. There isn't even a comparison between a person who has been cured of cancer, as against one who never had it. In contrast to some aspects of cancer therapy, where little can be done, an immense amount can be accomplished in cancer prevention. Strong anticigarette advertising legislation may have prevented many times the number of lung cancers than all of the physicians in the entire world will be able to cure in the next generation. In fact, anyone who has had any hand at all in inducing people to stop smoking can and should take credit for having prevented some deaths. I owe the fact that I stopped smoking, approximately fifteen years ago, to the statisticians that correlated smoking and lung cancer incidence and literally frightened me out of the habit— Thank you Drs. Doll, Hammond, Horn, et al.

There is no longer any doubt that x-irradiation and radiation produced by radioactive materials can cause leukemia, and a variety of other cancers. I repeat—there is no question that radiation produces cancer in man and animals. The only question that exists is, how much radiation does it take to produce a tumor of a specific type.

When I was considering obtaining a machine for irradiating mice, I considered the possibility of using a high voltage x-ray machine or the much cheaper cobalt source (some radioactive cobalt in a lead shield). I discussed the matter with our Radiation Safety Officer. He pointed out to me that you can always turn an x-ray machine off while the cobalt source continues to emit radiation. In case of an accident, the cobalt was potentially capable of doing much more damage. This comparison also holds for the pollution of our environment with radiation. When the amounts of medical and dental x-ray to which the population is exposed is reduced, the number of cancers caused by them will also go down. There is some indication that this decrease might already have started in the incidence of leukemia. In the last several years, the incidence of leukemia has actually gone down. There is some speculation that this might be due to the more judicious use of medical and dental x-ray—a plausible explanation. This is not likely to happen with regard to the radioactive isotopes that have entered the atmosphere as a result of atomic testing, and pollution of water and air by indiscriminate users of radioisotopes. Carbon is one of the building blocks of all living material, and carbon^{14} has a half-life of over 5,000 years. This means that of the radioactive carbon^{14} that is presently in our environment, half of it will still be around 5,000 years from now. This is a terrible legacy to leave those who will come after us. If we stop polluting the air with nonradioactive pollutants, it is a matter of time before most of these substances disappear from the environment—a relatively short time compared to how long it would take for the mass of radioactive isotopes to disappear. There is an interesting commentary about how our government functions: The National Cancer Institute is trying to prevent and cure cancer while the activities of the Atomic Energy Commission are instrumental in causing it.

It is noteworthy that the dread disease smallpox is still incurable—but it is no longer a serious problem in this country because it can be prevented.

It is, unfortunately, easier to get money to "cure" a disease than to "prevent" one.

The Mind and Cancer

Faith is a fine invention
For gentlemen who see;
But microscopes are prudent
In an emergency!

Emily Dickinson

The brain is connected to every part of the body by means of a network of nerves. These nerves carry signals from brain to body, and body to brain. Impulses coming to the brain are interpreted by the brain as touch, pain, pleasure, and so forth. If you hit your finger with a hammer, the finger does not feel the pain, the brain does; or if you wish, you do. A person with the nerves from the finger to the brain severed will not feel pain when the finger is injured. Since the brain is the "control center," everything that affects the body affects the brain and vice versa. Two aspirin tablets can have a profound effect upon how one feels without influencing the course of a disease. What aspirin does is effect the way that pain is either transmitted or perceived. Just as aspirin can attenuate pain and make one feel better, so can hypnotism, confidence in one's doctor, a zest for living, and a wide variety of things which effect the perception of pain and pleasure. Like aspirin, these mental states will probably not appreciably alter the course of a disease.

Much has been written about the importance of "a will to live." I know of no convincing objective evidence that a "will to live" can prolong life. The subjective findings that people with a "will to live" often live until the will to live disappears could just as easily be explained by postulating that this "will to live" merely vanishes with impending death. The "will to die" may be another story, and people who want to die may be able to bring it off by a variety of means. Children often believe that their thoughts can control life and death. They believe that if they wish someone dead that it will happen; and that if they wish it, they and others could live forever. Sometimes this fantasy gets into the medical literature disguised as science. I have to constantly guard against my own illusion of omnipotence and the fact that I tend to believe what I want to believe. There is a lot to be learned about mind over matter, and I am waiting for reliable data—not fantasy.

It is certain that a will to live and a zest for life affects the *quality* of one's life very profoundly. Whether or not it affects the *quantity* is a matter of conjecture.

Skillful psychotherapy can help incurably ill people, and their families, deal with illness and impending death, and can help people to more fully enjoy their remaining days together. Even people in the terminal stages of illness can be helped to feel better by using fantasy techniques, and by simply listening and conversing. When they are beyond benefiting from these things, then it is time for the physician's armamentarium of narcotizing drugs.

It is important to emphasize that there is nothing either new or magical about this and that it does not stop the course of the disease. No one has, to my knowledge, been cured of metastatic cancer by faith or psychotherapy. If it were possible, then psychiatrists would know how to live longer than the rest of us—and they haven't managed to do that (nor have faith healers).

Lung cancer may be preventable by anything which will induce someone not to smoke cigarettes. If psychologists and psychiatrists have an urge to "save lives," here might be a good place to start.

Since the quality of life may well be more important than its quantity, anything (and I do mean anything) that makes an incurably ill person feel better is a good thing. What I mean by "anything" includes psychotherapy, food, friendship, drugs, and so on. (I do not include things that hurt the survivors.)

The author of a recent best-selling book on psychology was quoted by a magazine as saying that "the treatment will work if the patient has faith in it." This is quite true; treatments in which faith is the only ingredient have been successful in making people feel better and in healing psychosomatic diseases. It is a good idea for the customer to shop around a bit, because the price of "faith" is quite variable. Some people do not believe that "cheap" faith can be as good as the high-priced variety. This is not true; the faith purchased by the wealthy is not a bit better than that purchased by the poor; in fact, the child who owns nothing usually has the best faith of all. There are often better remedies than faith: you don't have to have faith in penicillin or insulin or surgery for it to work. Faith should only be counted upon when all else has failed.

Fear

Many another, once, you schooled,
    giving strength to feeble hands;
    your words set right whoever wavered,
    and strengthened every failing knee.
And now your turn has come, and you
    lose patience too;
    now it touches you, and you are
    overwhelmed.

Job 4:3

Fear is something that we are all familiar with. It can be produced by a sudden noise in the middle of the night, or by a situation that is truly life-threatening. I remember one evening, about ten years ago, I was sitting and studying. I was pretty tired and, as I often do when I'm tired, started to rub the back of my neck. I felt a lump! I felt the other side and there was no such lump (I had been working with mouse Hodgkin's disease for over five years at that time, and often the first symptom of this disease is a lump in the neck). I shall never forget the terror. I went through the whole frightening process in my mind: the biopsy, the microscopic examination, the doctor saying that it was Hodgkin's disease, my getting other opinions to see if they could confirm it, deciding who to go to for treatment, what treatment to get? Nor shall I forget the relief, several days later, when a surgeon opened up my neck and told me that the tumor was a shiny bright yellow one, a lipoma (a fatty tumor that can usually be diagnosed by looking at it, and is almost always benign). When he removed the tumor and sewed up the incision, I danced out of the operating room—the weight of the world lifted from my shoulders. It was one of the happiest moments of my life.

The frequency of the occurrence of cancer is so high (about one person in four) that it is very hard to find a family in which at least one member has not been affected. The same is true of heart disease and stroke but, for some reason, cancer seems to be more terrifying to people than either heart disease or stroke. George Crile believes that this disproportionate fear has been induced by "those responsible for telling the public about cancer"—and I agree with him. People who daily take their lives into their hands on the nation's highways shudder at the mention of even the possibility that they might be harboring the seed of a cancer in their own body. I believe that an important element in the fear of cancer is a fear of the unknown. We are all more or less aware of the magnitude of the risk of accidental death on the highway, and can cope with it. Most people are able to accept the risk. They try to minimize it by being as careful as possible, and put it in the back of their minds along with such thoughts as the inevitability of death. Not so with cancer: A common attitude is that "If I have cancer, I don't want to know about it." It is, perhaps, the emotional equivalent of the young man who is so terrified of accidental death that he courts it by driving his car in excess of 100 miles an hour—see, you can't hurt me! As with automobile accidents, much can be done to reduce the risk; while nothing can be done to eliminate the risk. Most tumors, but not all, grow slowly for a period of time before they spread. If they can be removed surgically at this time, the patient is cured.

There are some risks which are exceptionally high among certain groups of people. The person who is (or was) a heavy smoker would do well to obtain a complete physical annually, including a chest x-ray.

The most careful driver can have a tire blowout on a highway and be killed, but the probability of being killed on the highway is less to the careful driver than the careless one. The same is true of the risk of dying of cancer. You may know someone who died of lung cancer and never smoked; by the same token, you might also know someone who won the Irish Sweepstakes. In other words, it is possible to reduce the risk of getting lung cancer. I hope that reducing the objective risk might also reduce the subjective fear. I used to worry about getting lung cancer. Instead of trying to reduce the worry, I reduced the risk by giving up the weed. Since I quit smoking fifteen years ago, lung cancer no longer worries me.

While there have been changes in the treatment of disease, the ways that physician and patient approach one another has not changed. People still come to their physicians frightened and hope that he can alleviate their fears. The woman whose parents both succumbed to heart attacks wants to be told that her heart is in good shape, while the man who has lost a parent to cancer wants to be told that he does not have cancer. This need for consolation is intensified by people being bombarded with advertising that tells them how fearful cancer and heart disease is. While patients are becoming more fearful, physicians are becoming less personal and less able to deal with the fears. Anyone who has gone to a busy physician recently has probably found that the doctor has little time for feelings because he is too busy with seriously ill people who require that he minister to their physical needs. The physician who was the family friend, father confessor, and general purveyor of comfort has all but disappeared. Most people have a need to have someone to tell their troubles to. If this is a problem with relatively healthy people, think of how terrible it must be to someone who is facing death.

There is a public outcry for a return to the days when the physician was a friend of the family and not only helped them medically, but comforted them emotionally. In this mobile society in which we live, it is unlikely that we will ever recreate the old country doctor. Besides, I don't think that we would really want to. The old country doctor was very good at comforting the sick and dying, but he was damned ineffective in actually curing disease. We need all of the help that scientific medicine can provide. There is, however, nothing in scientific medicine that is incompatible with the physician also being humane. Dr. Elisabeth Kubler-Ross would like the physician to be able to handle both the physical and the emotional aspects of patient care. Her goal is a laudable one which might be attainable with many physicians, but certainly not with all of them. This is what the thinking medical educator would build into all of his physicians if he could. The ideal physician understands scientific medicine (what medical science can and cannot do for a patient) and also can comfort his patients when he can do no more for them physically. It is also what every patient wants in a physician.

No one person can be expected to do everything. The man who performs the surgery may be temperamentally unsuited to provide the emotional support his patient may need; and by the same token the person able to provide the emotional support may be incapable of performing the surgery. Some psychiatrists have assumed the role of helping the incurably ill, as have many ministers. There are not enough professionals available to handle the problem. Besides, psychiatrists, like surgeons, also find themselves swamped with the seriously mentally ill and do not have time to comfort the dying. It seems to me that the only solution to the problem is the education of everyone in desirable ways of dying—and living.

When a doctor tells you, or someone you love, that you have cancer it's as if you just had your death warrant signed. There is no escaping the terror. As Elisabeth Kubler-Ross describes it, the first reaction is usually "This couldn't be happening to me." This is followed by anger, with the "victim" resenting everyone else who is healthy, and wondering what they could have done to deserve this. This stage is magnificently described in the book of Job. Following this comes a stage of acceptance in which a person is ready to deal with reality. Fortunately, in most cases, the realities are nowhere near as grim as the word "cancer" implies. Many cases can be completely cured with surgery and the patient with incurable cancer often has many pain-free years before the end.

One of the most difficult things that a person with cancer

has to deal with is the fact that there can never be certainty. One is never sure whether the operation has actually cured the disease or not. Even if the operation did not cure the disease, or the disease was untreatable, one has no idea whether the end will come soon, or not for many years. The nagging problem is this uncertainty. It might be easier to live with the certainty of immediate impending death, than it is not to know how long. Yet, we all of us have to handle the fact that very few things in life are "certain." There are dangers inherent in driving a car, swimming, riding a bicycle, or even walking on the streets. The person who is aware of this uncertainty nevertheless makes some adjustments to it. Most of us proceed with some illusion of certainty, because it is the only practical thing to do. To do otherwise is to live in constant terror. Most of us are able to utilize illusion when it is necessary to do so. For most of our lives, we act as if we were, in fact, immortal. The diagnosis of cancer says something to you that you have been aware of for a long time— that you are going to die, but you don't know when. You have been aware of it, but have ignored it. Most reasonable people look at the grim realities for a while, and then reestablish their illusion of immortality. Even people with incurable cancer usually have a number of years in which they are feeling well and in which they can do anything that people without cancer can do. Some people with incurable cancer have managed to accept it, and have made their remaining years rich and meaningful for themselves and the people around them. Others have frozen the rest of their lives in the panic stage, and have spent their remaining time desperately searching for cures that did not exist. They have essentially managed to die emotionally at the time of the diagnosis. They were deprived of many years of effective living.

If you have been diagnosed as having cancer, you would be well advised to first get the best possible treatment that is available and to then go on living as best you can. Every year that passes without a sign of recurrence means that the chances of your having been cured by the treatment are better and, by five years for most curable cancers, you are pretty well out of the woods. In the meantime, you have not wasted what may well be one-fifth to one-twentieth of your life stewing about the possibility that you are going to die.

The same basic approach is useful should you find out that you have an incurable type of cancer for which medical science can do nothing or at best prolong your life by a few years. People who have been able to resign themselves to a limited life have been able to make their remaining time as rich and meaningful as possible for both themselves and their loved ones. I strongly recommend that, should you find yourself in this predicament, you read Elisabeth Kubler-Ross' book called *On Death and Dying.* You may find this hard to believe, but some people with incurable cancer have made the last few years of their life the most meaningful and beautiful ones for both themselves and the people around them.

There is another general rule for successful living that is particularly useful to people with incurable cancer: it is *DON'T LOOK BACK.* It does little good to stew about the things that you might have done, or should not have done.

To Tell the Truth

Trying to conceal the truth about cancer from the patient is like trying to hide an elephant under the living room rug.

What makes the tragedy of concealment ironic is that no one has ever succeeded in doing it. I have seen a husband trying to conceal the truth from his wife while she is trying not to reveal that she knows the truth. The amount of energy wasted in this futile deception could be spent in the couple supporting one another in a myriad of ways. Instead of helping each other to face their respective losses, many people (and their physicians) try to conceal the truth. To lie successfully under these circumstances is something that a professional actor would have trouble with; yet doctors and wives and husbands delude themselves with the thought that they are really carrying it off.

There are very few things that I am sure of—one of them is that concealing the truth from an adult with incurable cancer is usually disastrous. There is no point in the macabre conspiracy of silence. The patient knows, or can guess, how ill he is; this being the case all of the efforts at concealment are wasted. Added to this is the patient's feeling that there is no one whom he can trust and talk to; and that he has to protect those around him from the truth that they are protecting him from (sic) a truly Gordian Laingian knot. The consequences of concealment are more pain rather than less and considerably less love and comfort for everyone involved.

I do not mean that the truth should be forced upon

someone. When a person is ready for the truth, he will ask. When he does ask, he should be told the complete truth—and there should be a loving shoulder nearby to cry on. Who does the telling depends upon who is able to. If possible someone should be on hand who has accurate information, but it is not necessary. The important thing is to have someone who cares. I have seen whole families handle the problem together, and all have been drawn closer to one another as a consequence.

People who faced impending death openly found that their remaining time together was among their best, while those who concealed were continually fearful lest "he should find out." One would think that not being too close would make the parting easier (if you're farther apart you won't care so much) but it doesn't; it only adds an additional burden of guilt for not having done more to make the patient's remaining days happier. It is so much better to tell someone that you love him and don't want him to die, than to have to say it years later to an empty chair in a Gestalt therapy session.

There is one more important reason to make it a policy to tell the truth. If someone does *not* have cancer, they will believe you instead of wondering what is being concealed.

The relationship between patient and doctor can also be an open and honest one. I believe that the most rewarding relationship between patient and doctor is one where the patient is treated as the equal of the physician in everything but the physician's professional expertise. In short, the doctor should treat his patient with the same respect that he expects from his automobile mechanic. On this basis, the patient may be able to make both an intelligent and informed decision about his own life.

The physicians I have known whose professional activities have enriched their own lives have been those who prefer this way of dealing with their patients. Making life and death decisions for others can lead to many a sleepless night, while helping others to make their own decisions can be very gratifying. Doctors who perpetually make decisions *for* others are often continually agitated and spend the better part of their lives running—from office to hospital to golf course and back again.

Forgiving

I remember every harsh word I said to her in those years. And though reason tells me that they came simply from strain and were inevitable, I have tried to take them back a hundred times, to ask forgiveness. But I am not forgiven. The survivor is the sinner and cannot forgive himself, and the only person who could forgive is gone.

Robert Anderson, *After*

Whenever someone dies, the people left behind often feel responsible, in some way, for their death. Remarks that begin with "If only I had . . ." or "I should have . . ." testify to that guilt. Sometimes the guilt can be crippling. If the person who is dying forgives their loved ones for their real and imagined sins, the subsequent adjustment to the loss can be made immeasurably easier.

Some kind of guilt is virtually guaranteed because the survivor almost always resents the person he loves for leaving (deserting) him. As a child is angry when his mother "goes away," so does an adult feel about the loss of someone close, such as a spouse or parent or child. In the middle of this anger at being deserted is the thought that he has no right to be angry because the other person is suffering more than he is and, besides, is not responsible for what is happening. If the anger is verbalized and the survivor is absolved of guilt for his feelings, it goes a long way toward his eventual recovery. It helps both the survivor and the dying person if they are aware of the mixed feelings that invariably exist.

Anger is as natural as love, and is always present in any crisis. If it is dealt with openly and intelligently, it can be dissipated where it will do no harm. Anger is like gunpowder: in the open it burns; when tightly enclosed, it explodes— with unpredictable results.

For the dying person, the present time is all that he has, but the person who will live on has a future to be concerned with. He may have to take care of small' children, comfort others, and make all kinds of necessary arrangements. While the present is equally important to him, he must also be concerned about the future. The resolution (closure) of one's affairs with the dying person is important, and can minimize guilt which will add to the inevitable pain. Cancer is a disease which allows this resolution. In contrast, sudden death often leaves people without an opportunity to say good-by properly —it leaves people feeling unfinished. It is sometimes an emotional disaster for the survivor if someone dies suddenly, during or after what would ordinarily be a trivial quarrel.

Before my brother died, he wrote the following:

THOUGHTS AND STUFF
by Eli Pilgrim

It is customary, I guess, in a time like this to leave some words behind.

First, I want to put the responsibility of dying (it's hard to write that word) on no one. I want no one to feel he could have done something—not relatives, friends, doctors. I don't even put the blame on (for those who may believe in Him) God.

I can't say I like the situation. I have regrets leaving before some dreams come true. I did want to see Haley's Comet and the 21st Century.

To all my friends I say thanks for the pinochle and company. I'm sorry I had to beat you so often.

To Ira and Jean, thanks I can't express. I've known you both a very short time, but you have added something to my life that made it more complete. I wish I could write in detail, but I never could go on-and-on on a subject. I know you have a wonderful life ahead. Wish I were there.

(I should be careful in writing all this stuff because a misplaced word could make a difference.)

I have no last requests. I have thought of giving my body to some school, but I don't know yet.

It's so damn hard to write of these things.

I want no big headstone. Maybe plant a tree instead. Maybe I'll think of a brilliant epitaph.

Mom and Dad, I love you both very much and don't want you to feel that any of this is in any way your fault. Nothing you could have done would have made any difference.

My personal property has been taken care of. My retirement fund with the University goes to Mom and Dad.

I'll edit this tomorrow and brush up the lousy sentence structure and sloppy handwriting, made sloppier because I am lying down.

Tomorrow never came for Eli.

His letter made things easier for all of us.

I don't know what it is like to die. That is something that can be experienced only once—there are no experts. I do know what it feels like to lose someone I love—I have experienced that too many times. The pain lasts for a long time.

I would welcome knowing in advance when I am about to die, because I would like to do for those who survive me what those who loved me and died did for me.

On Impending Death

(For people who have incurable cancer
and for those who love them.)

Today you've got the strength of a bull in your neck
And the strength of a bear in your arms,
But some o' these days, some o' these days,
You'll have a hand-to-hand struggle with bony Death,
And Death is bound to win.

James Weldon Johnson,
"The Prodigal Son" in *God's Trombones*

There is little that I can say to someone who is facing impending death that will ease his burden. I usually come back to what my father used to say to me (and what I now tell my children) when I was faced with an impossible and painful situation. He would tell me "Yes, it's terrible and it hurts—but that's the way it is."

I have given a lot of thought to how one deals with death. I always come back to the same conclusion: you do not deal with death—death deals with you. I conclude that, since there is no way of avoiding the tragedy, then one might as well do a good job of dying. As Shakespeare said,

And nothing 'gainst Time's scythe can make defence
Save breed, to brave him when he takes thee hence.

It has been a long time since the first person who was dear to me died. I tried to escape. I have since learned to deal with death and dying. I no longer run, because I know that running only makes the pain last longer and adds guilt to the pain. I know that I can do something to make it easier for the person I love and for me—I have learned to comfort others and myself.

A parent can make his child feel better, when he is hurting, with a kiss, a band-aid, a pat on the head, and words of comfort. Since, psychologically, hurt seems to happen to the "child" part of the self, the same things can be done for an adult. While the grown-up child is treated somewhat differently, the same principles apply. Gently massaging a person's body does wonders for the patient—and the therapist. Words of love and comfort also help, but touching seems to feel better. For some, a shoulder to cry on and someone who cares goes a long way toward relieving anguish.

Georg Groddeck says,

> A yearning is in me: when I am sad my heart cries for my mother, and she is not to be found. Am I then to grumble at God's world? Better to laugh at myself, at this childishness from which we never emerge, for never do we quite grow up; we manage it rarely, and then only on the surface; we merely play at being grown up as a child plays at being big. So soon as we live intensely we become children. . . . Do but look upon someone in his moments of deepest sorrow . . . his eyes glisten or cloud over. . . . No one cries any more after he is grown up? But that is only because it is not the custom, because some silly idiot or other sent it out of fashion.*

The long-lasting pain is reserved for those who are left behind. The dying person has his moment of agony and then it is over. The people left behind feel the loss for much of their lives.

Life holds two great terrors: one is the terror of ME dying and the other is the terror of losing someone whom I love. Both the terror and the attendant grief are things that do not happen to "other people," but to the self. When my father died, I wept mostly for ME. I cried because I was lonely and I knew that I would never again hear his voice or feel

* Groddeck, Georg, *The Book of the It*, page 20 (New York: New American Library, Mentor Books, 1961).

his touch. For me, the world was a lonelier and diminished place when he left it. I was also aware that HE was not in pain.

I have learned to cope with death and dying. Regrettably, I am almost getting to be proficient at it. I suppose that I shall have to deal with death several more times before my own turn comes to die. Dealing with death is the part of life which I find the most painful—yet, I would rather be the person who has to deal with death than be the one experiencing it.

Many people have pointed out that it is important for people to say their "good-bys." Why it is important is hard to define except to point out that people who do not say their good-bys are profoundly troubled by it for a long time.

After someone dies the only way of venting grief is to "cry it out." Again, there is only the empiric observation that people who do not vent their grief are troubled with it for a longer time than those who do. In contrast to people who do not mourn, who carry the scars of death with them for a long time, those who do mourn find that after a time the grief is replaced by wistful memories.

I have dealt with the death of someone dear to me by running away from it and by facing it directly and dealing with it. The effect of running was emotional disaster. All of the people I know who have dealt with death and dying agree that facing it and mourning is far better than avoiding it; and that the price of avoidance and denial is, in the long run, a much greater one.

L'Envoi

Now it is said:
The words to unerasable printer's ink committed;
And I have done
What I feared most to do;
Put on clinician's mantle,
Knowing that by so doing
I both preserve and kill;
That where I am in error,
Or not clear,
Someone may die sooner
Because of words I wrote.

I apologize to myself and say
"That for the love of those in pain,
I use the power of the pen
To give some comfort;
Help some to see what choices are."
And know this is not true—
I write from vanity,
And hope that I am wise enough
To give more comfort than pain
—More life than death.

I have tried, insofar as it is possible, to keep this part of the book general, and have avoided being too specific. My reason for doing this is that information changes, and often very rapidly. I do not want to tout a particular treatment only to find that the information is wrong. What I have said and documented about breast cancer applies equally well, in principle, to most other forms of cancer and their treatment. It should give a patient some idea about the questions they might ask their physicians, and roughly how much salt should be taken with the answers. There is no way that I know of to provide specific answers based on generalities. Nor can anyone predict what will happen to an individual by looking at the odds.

It is extremely difficult to maintain one's rationality in the face of the most severe emotional stress imaginable—impending death. Hopefully, the reader in these straits has already selected a physician who is basically a rational man. The rational physician has learned to cope with many of the problems of the cancer patient. He is also a human being, and has his "hang-ups."

As in most human transactions there is a lot to be gained from all parties having a high degree of awareness. I know of no easy way to acquire this, and often it is in the process of handling difficult situations that the awareness comes—sometimes too late to be of much value.

I think that I have probably been too hard on the surgeon and therapists. This was deliberate, because I think that the types of inquiries that this book provokes will eventually help both the physician and the patient. I hope that the love and compassion that I feel for the conscientious physician has not been obscured by our differences. I believe that the physician is basically "good," even though the results of some of the things that he does may be "bad." Mistakes have to be considered in the light of the amount of comfort that the physician gives to the patients; and one must always be aware that he is often forced to make decisions based on entirely inadequate information. He is not someone apart—he is in the same boat that the rest of us are in.

Virtually all of the undesirable things that are done in the world are done by good, well-meaning people. I have only to think of the people whom I have injured, and to conjecture about the potential effects of this book, to know that I am not someone apart. I have taken R. D. Laing's advice and looked at myself in a mirror. What I see there is at least as disturbing to me as what I see elsewhere. I do not wish to criticize people, only acts; and to increase the accuracy of the information available to the public. I regret that I could not provide the definitive information that many of you need in order to make rational decisions. Some of the information is accessible to your physician; but most of the important data just does not exist at the present time.

PART IV

CANCER POLITICS

"But I don't want to go among mad people," Alice remarked.

"Oh, you can't help that," said the Cat: "We're all mad here. I'm mad. You're mad."

"How do you know I'm mad?" said Alice.

"You must be," said the Cat, "or you wouldn't have come here."

Lewis Carroll, *Alice's Adventures in Wonderland*

The Cancer Cure Con

C Y N I C , n. A blackguard whose faulty vision sees things as they are, not as they ought to be. Hence the custom among the Scythians of plucking out a cynic's eyes to improve his vision.

Ambrose Bierce, *The Devil's Dictionary*

In 1889 Dr. Roswell Park made this proposal to the New York State Legislature: If they would give him $10,000, within two years he would find the cure for cancer. The State Legislature gave him the money at a time when New York State did not even have a state-supported system for higher education. As it exists today, the Roswell Park Institute itself contains many dedicated scientists and physicians and is now part of the State University system. In this capacity, its contribution to the general welfare of the state has increased more than enough to justify the expenditure and its existence. My dispute is not with the Institute as it exists today, but with the premise on which it was founded.

The classic confidence, or con game, is selling the Brooklyn Bridge to the newly arrived immigrant or visitor. It is extracting money for something that cannot possibly be delivered, because the person doing the selling does not have it to deliver. Selling the Brooklyn Bridge is an obvious swindle. There also seems to be no question about the immorality of selling someone a cancer cure that doesn't work. But what if the personal gain isn't obvious, and the promise is made "in good faith"—is it any less of a con? Isn't it also a con to say to the public "If you will give me so much money, I promise to find a cure for cancer"? The "con" becomes more obvious if you contrast it to the kinds of statements that would be made by the honest scientist. He tells his patrons that he is going to spend his time trying to find a cure, or trying to discover the cause. He is promising to deliver only his time and effort—and that he can deliver! He may express optimism; and that is only natural. No one drops a fishing line in a pond unless he thinks that there are fish in it.

Dr. Roswell Park's logical descendants are still operating, but they no longer ask for $10,000. The figure runs into the millions. They may command a favorable press, which often states, in one way or another, that the cure for cancer is just around the corner. While hope springs eternal, there is no scientific basis for such unbridled optimism. The cancer problem is nowhere near as simple as the problem of poliomyelitis; and while there have been some notable victories (some effective surgical, x-ray, and chemical treatments for cancer) it still promises to be a long, uphill struggle.

I have been asked if my attitude would be different if Dr. Park had actually been successful and found the cure for cancer. My answer is that it certainly would be different. But he didn't discover the cure for cancer, and the probability of his discovering it was much slimmer then than it is now—and at the present time it's a long shot. What is important is that there is a limit to the amount of money that can be spent on cancer, and it should be spent where it will do the most good.

Most of us have some bias about how important intentions are. Some people are willing to forgive anything if intentions are good, and some people are willing to overlook almost anything if the result is good, caring little about what motivated the action. Whenever a child is accidentally struck by an automobile there are people who would gladly hang the driver, and others who would forgive him, saying that he is suffering enough for what he has done. As anyone who has studied the problem of capital punishment knows, there are some very powerful arguments on both sides. There are no easy decisions where life and death are involved, and I would not be discussing Dr. Roswell Park if it wasn't for the fact that the same arguments that he used in 1889 are being used today in attempts to extract money from the American public.

I do not know, nor could I even venture a guess to say where and when the discoveries which we consider to be major breakthroughs may occur. I do not even know in what field they will occur. They might occur in the field of industrial plastics, for all I know. Increased probability of success (and a maximum utilization of funds) lies with the support of intelligent, imaginative people who will use the funds in attempts to find the answers to important problems. It does not seem improbable to me to think that the not-too-distant future will supply many of the answers to problems of differentiation, the way that the gene acts, the way that cancer spreads, and how cells can tell friends from enemies. Yet, when someone makes the statement, "The cancer problem will be solved in the next ten years," I check to see if my wallet is still in my pocket. These statements are as unwarranted now as they were 50 years ago, or 100 years ago, or 1,000 years ago, for that matter. Translated into business terms, it is a promise to parlay one dollar into a million in a few years—an obvious swindle.

I don't wish to leave the impression that anyone who is interested in curing or preventing cancer is a con artist. There are people and agencies doing their work both quietly and noisily, who are not attempting to hoodwink the public. Nor do I wish to imply that what I've referred to as the "cancer cure con" is a *conscious* effort to deception. It is often the result of people with very deep emotional commitments to the cure of cancer who let their pen and tongue get carried away. Many actually believe that the cure is just around the corner.

I am aware that attacking what I call the cancer cure con is heresy. To say that it is fundamentally dishonest to promise something that cannot be delivered is to attack the very roots of our culture. The business ethic states that the most important thing is to "sell the product." If the product falls apart once the money is collected, it is often considered to be a bigger "score." The rationale for producing products that do not fall apart is that, if the product is good the next sale will be easier. The business ethic also pervades medicine and science. There are honest scientists, just as there are honest businessmen. These honest people are rarely successful in the short pull, but they are sometimes listened to when people become totally disillusioned with the con men. I would like to see the science deck stacked in favor of the honest man.

At the present time the scientist has some grace that the businessman does not have. The public is still willing to listen, and believe what the scientist says. That grace is not likely to last very long if the "Roswell Parks" are allowed to have their way.

The Cancer Buck

To understand how the federal cancer budget works, try taking your household budget and moving each decimal point
six to eight spaces to the right. Then round everything off to
the nearest million.

In the late 1930s, the Federal Government entered the cancer
research business. The National Cancer Institute started with a
total budget of $400,000 (it's now $400,000,000). This budget
supported the beginnings of the National Cancer Institute in
Bethesda, Maryland; about $100,000 supported research proj-
ects, and $8,000 was devoted to research fellowships and train-
ing grants (combined).

The advent of World War II eliminated the possibility of
the expansion of cancer research, and the status quo was
barely maintained. Immediately following the end of the war,
there was an increase in federal spending (presumably to keep
the economy from being inundated) and a substantial segment
of this went into cancer research, with a logarithmic increase
in the amount of the budget for the National Cancer Institute
into the tens of millions of dollars. The budget for cancer research, aside from a small slump in the early 1950s, continued
to increase under the Eisenhower administration, although at
a slower rate. Had it continued at the same rate as it had in the
previous four years, it would have occupied the entire federal
budget, and there would have been no money left for anything

else. (Remember the chapter on growth?) We might not even have been able to afford a war in Southeast Asia. The Kennedy administration had little added effect on cancer research.* The Johnson and Nixon Administrations not only leveled the budget for cancer research, but did not allow enough of an increase to take care of the decreased value of the dollar due to inflation. While the graphs may look as if they have leveled off, funds available for noncontract cancer research have gone steadily downhill since 1963.

There is nothing secret about where the money appropriated for the National Cancer Institute goes. It is all published in a pamphlet called National Cancer Institute Fact Book which is published by the institute itself and can be obtained by writing for it. This pamphlet is a breakdown of the organization of the institute and where the money goes.

In 1956 Congress thought that it was time for chemical warfare on cancer—to cure it, that is; and the Cancer Chemotherapy Program was started. This was the beginning of the institute's contract research program. It set the stage for the massive contract programs to come. Research contracts cost 82 million dollars in 1971, and were budgeted at 138 million for 1973, which is more than is spent for the research grants program, which finances cancer research in the entire nation. It is ten times the amount spent for fellowships and training grants.

One of the major budget categories is called "Collaborative Research and Development." This massive program includes most of the research that is directly controlled by the National Cancer Institute. It includes research that is done at the institute itself, and research contracted out. About 85% of the budget for "Collaborative Research and Development" represents research contracts.

* About a year after the Kennedy administration started, I was talking to a friend who had an administrative post with the National Science Foundation. I asked him how the "New Frontier" was treating science. He said, "When we sent our budget to the Eisenhower administration, we were told that we had to economize and would get a 10% increase. When we send our budget to the Kennedy administration, we are told that the administration is all for science and wanted to do everything that it can—there would be a 10% increase."

There is no question about where the major financial support has been going in the last five or ten years, and where it is still going. It is going to support research controlled directly from Bethesda, Maryland, via the contract program, and to support large cancer institutes. The distribution of grant funds pretty much parallels the distribution of cancer research scientists. Large amounts go to California where there are a number of large university centers; Illinois, which reflects concentration of medical and scientific talent around Chicago; Massachusetts, which has a considerable amount of medical and research talent concentrated around Boston. The same is true of New York, Pennsylvania, and Texas.

With research contracts, the same thing applies. Those states having large numbers of cancer research scientists also receive contracts as well as grants. In contrast, there is a group of states clustered around Bethesda—from whence comes the control—which receive most of the contract money. This includes Maryland (which receives the lion's share of the contract money), the District of Columbia, and Virginia. In fact, the specifications on some contracts read that the installation cannot be more than a certain distance from Bethesda. In short, there is a relationship between proximity to Bethesda and the awarding of contracts. It is interesting that the National Cancer Institute prefers to refer to these contracts as something separate from the growth of the institute itself. While it is physically separate, it does, nonetheless, represent a massive growth of the federal bureaucracy.

In 1971 Congress added one hundred million dollars to the budget of the National Cancer Institute. Where did that one hundred million go? Did it go toward reviving the foundering cancer research programs in the nation that were funded by grants? Did it go to support independent creative scientists? No! Most of it went into the contract program. The research grant program received an additional ten million dollars (an additional 15 percent) which was not enough to restore the grant program to its preinflation level; and ended up by putting only half of that into the hands of the scientists, after overhead and other expenses had been taken out. It didn't even take care of inflated costs. Another $26 million went to cancer research centers, which again support large programs. The largest single amount of money went to Collaborative Research and Development Program ($58 million), which increases its financing by almost 60 percent.

Along with the working scientists, cancer institutes were also hurting. Most of these institutes operate on grant and contract money. People who run cancer institutes, in contrast to working scientists, are highly influential—so, the first commitment of the new "cancer crusade" was to the cancer institutes. It is a political axiom that you never ask for money for yourself; you ask for money for a national program. If it goes through, you end up with your share. Therefore, instead of looking for money to support the existing cancer institutes, what was asked for was the creation of a group of new cancer institutes. There are barely enough scientists, cancer physicians, and so on to staff the existing institutes. Yet, this was the first place to get money when the increased cancer budget came through.

At the same time that the amount of money appropriated for Cancer Research was going up, the actual amount that was getting to the cancer scientist to pay for his equipment, technicians, and so forth was rapidly decreasing. It was decreasing because of inflation (which everybody knows about) and because overhead costs had skyrocketed. Overhead is essentially the cost of doing business that is not measured by direct expenditures. An oversimplified example would be the cost of maintaining a heating plant, electricity, janitorial service, a personnel department. Some industries charge the government overhead costs of 150 to 300 percent, and I have been told that the actual overhead in university operations approaches 85 percent of the cost of salaries and fringe benefits.

I would like to make the categorical statement that much of the present cost of overhead in university-conducted research is superfluous, and much has been created to satisfy the arbitrary needs of the federal bureaucracy. University administrations are continually crying that the overhead rates do not pay for the cost of doing research—that they are (sob) losing money. All this in the face of the following facts: (1) The administrative structures of all institutions that receive substantial amounts of grant and contract funds have not only increased in size, but some have become downright plush. (2) A large number of the people employed by these institutions have their time paid for, either in part or in full, by federal funds. (3) Organizations whose sole function is the procurement of government money now exist in universities as well as in industry. (4) Administrative faculty members (heads of departments, and so on) are often hired for their ability to acquire grants and contracts. If universities are losing money on research, how come a major part of their endeavor is devoted to attracting more government money? When overhead rates were considerably less than what they are now, universities were working hard at obtaining government grants and contracts because there was (you should excuse the expression) profit * in it. Fortunately, when overhead rates were low, they could not put the amount of money into the procurement of contracts that they now do.

My reason for attacking this aspect of fiscal policy is because it has taken money out of the hands of the scientists and placed it elsewhere. *If the federal government allocated a certain amount of money to cancer research scientists and then a separate amount of money to overhead, the disparity would become very apparent to the public. Instead it is all lumped in one category.* Appropriations for the National Cancer Institute have gone up by $40 million in the last five years. In the face of these hard statistics, it is extremely difficult to convince the public that the amount of money given to cancer research scientists to do cancer research has gone down. The amount of money allocated to research grants has gone up from about $70 million in 1965 to about $95 million in 1970. This is a 36 percent increase in five years. At the same time, overhead costs have increased by 50 percent and the cost of equipment and salaries have also increased considerably.

There are many things that industry can do better than universities or research institutes. However, I find myself

---

* I am using the word "profit" in its actual sense, not its legalistic one. Profit can be measured in many ways besides money. A nonprofit institution has buildings, offices, equipment, travel expenses, pays salaries (sometimes very large ones)—in short, it does not do what it does for love.

somewhat skeptical about the efficacy of industries that continually require, not only priming, but complete government support. The argument has been raging, for as far back as I can remember, about the relative efficacy of the free enterprise system (capitalism) versus planned economy (socialism). Unfortunately, compromises between the two often result in neither free enterprise nor planned economy. What is usually incorporated are the worst features of the two systems rather than the best. In the industries that are supported by contracts, we have "free enterprise" under "complete government control." I would like to suggest the term "freak enterprise." So far as I can tell there is nothing free about them, and the only "enterprise" involved is an ability to acquire government money.

I have been well taught about the necessity for free competition, and I believe it. I have also been taught that planning is desirable, and I believe that too. The idea that it is possible to effectively combine the two is something I do not believe. With regard to science, it seems desirable to have both systems existing side by side—but not together. We can have research in private industry, research in universities, research in government installations, and research by private individuals. The danger in the current trends of federal support for research (contracts) is that all of these diverse ways of doing things will eventually become one, and scientific creativity may be stifled.

The National Cancer Institute has expanded far beyond anything that its founders ever dreamed of. I am sure that at that time there must have been some who were well enough versed in the politics to predict that you can't have pork without pigs. It is a basic fact of politics (human nature, if you wish) that every time there is a pot of gold there will be people who will try to get it. There is nothing about science or medicine that confers an immunity to avarice. What keeps men from being excessively greedy is the fact that grabbing too much often results in a rap on the knuckles by others who also want their share. Politicians are used to thinking in terms of the pork barrel, while scientists are not. Scientists are not used to thinking in these terms because, until recently, there has never been very much pork in the barrel, and what there was had to be divided up in some reasonable way. This has changed since World War II, and an excellent account of how it has changed can be found in Daniel Greenberg's book *The Politics of Pure Science*—a book that made Greenberg as popular with big science as Ralph Nader was with General Motors.

Research Grants vs. Research Contracts

> There is something self-defeating about scientists being owned, or managed, or directed. The essence of creativity is rebellion and independence. The type of individual who will allow himself to be directed is probably incapable of any large measure of creativity. The creative scientist will either be stifled or will go to some other line of work which allows him to be independent.

There are two routes through which a scientist can obtain money to finance his research: the grant system and the contract system.

The research grant system is the principal route that scientists outside of government go through to obtain funds. All of the branches of the National Institutes of Health, including the National Cancer Institute, use the research grant system. This method is also used by the National Science Foundation and by a number of private agencies. A grant proposal is initiated by the scientist and is sent to the proper agency. From there the proposal goes to a study section. The study section consists of scientists drawn from all parts of the country, who are specialists in the field. They review the application and either approve or reject it. If they approve it, it is given a priority number which will determine whether or not it is funded if there is a limited amount of money. A high priority usually guarantees that the money will be available, and a low priority means that the money will not be forthcoming if there is not enough money available. Often the people on the study section are familiar with the professional competence of the applicant, and have some idea of the feasibility of the project. Ten years ago almost any well-trained beginning scientist was able to get money to do his research. Today, study sections are much more selective, and tend not to support either the young beginning scientist nor projects that appear to be a long shot.

Study sections may be thought of as self-perpetuating bodies. The members of the section either pick their successors, or have a good deal to say about who their successors should be.

This peer review system has certain advantages and disadvantages. On the debit side, it might be said that the people that staff the study sections represent scientific orthodoxy, and that they would tend to downgrade highly imaginative projects. To its credit, it is a system that is far better than anything that has been devised so far. It is as good, or imaginative, as the men that staff the study sections. This problem of the relative lack of grant support of imaginative projects is not entirely the fault of the people on the study sections. With increased public pressures for "results," and a shortage of money, it is only natural that study sections would tend to support the safe bets. When money is more available, there is more of a tendency for the members of the study sections to say "Let's take a chance." Many risky projects have been financed. A good example of a "take a chance" project is the type that would allow a new Ph.D. like James Watson to take a trip to Europe to see what was going on. We are too close to the events of the day to be able to see which discoveries will be important in the future and which will not. It is, however, safe to say that most projects, at the time that they are initially proposed, are highly uncertain. I wonder how some of the following proposals, which are now proved successes, would fare in today's research grant climate: (1) A proposal to explore the natural populations of animals on certain islands (Charles Darwin). (2) A proposal to investigate whether organisms that cannot be seen can cause disease (Pasteur). (3) An investigation of the effect of physicians washing their hands on the occurrence of child-bed fever (Semmelweis). (4) A study of sex and neurosis (Freud).

There is a happy middle ground that will support many sound projects and a few that have a marginal probability of success. It is possible to err too much on one side and support every crackpot proposal that is submitted; but it is equally undesirable to only support those that have a very high chance of success.

From the study section the application goes to The National Advisory Cancer Council. The council is comprised of men of considerable stature—whatever that means. They generally approve the recommendations of the study section, but sometimes overrule it. The council is the highest court of appeals that a scientist has, but it is rarely used in this way.

If the scientist gets his money, he goes to work. He is required to submit an annual progress report to the institute, and to supply reprints of his publications. Grants are approved for varying periods of time ranging from one to seven years, and at the end of that time the scientist again finds himself in competition with other scientists for the renewal of his grant.

The other source of support is the research contract.* There are other types of government contracts which involve the production of animals, or special reagents, or building facilities. I am not going to be concerned with these, but will devote the entire discussion to the "research contract."

In contrast to the research grant, the research contract proposal is usually initiated by the government. The federal planners decide that a certain type of research should be done, and they advertise for a contractor in an appropriate publication. Sometimes the proposal is initiated by the scientist himself, who will ask a government agency if it is interested in giving him a contract to do something that he thinks they might want done. An important distinction between the grant and contract system is that in the contract system it is manda-

---

* The people in Bethesda refer to the work that is done inside of the Cancer Institute and the work that is contracted out as "inhouse" and "outhouse" research.

tory that "the government" be interested in what the scientist wants to do. If, for example, a scientist were interested in studying how cells move around in the body, he would not apply for a contract with the cancer chemotherapy people because this would probably not be the type of work that they were interested in having done. If, on the other hand, he was interested in testing a new drug that he had discovered, that might have some possibilities as a chemotherapeutic agent, the contract route might be a reasonable way to proceed.

The usual way that contracts are developed is for the government agency to propose, in a general way, what they want done; and have the scientist submit a project proposal on how he wished to do it. Often, the proposal is worked out by the representatives of the agency and the scientist together. The proposal is reviewed by the agency and approved. Since the people reviewing it have had a hand in its preparation, it is not too likely that a proposal will be rejected. Sometimes competitive proposals are submitted; and in that case the agency has to choose between competing proposals to do the same job. In these cases, there is a review in fact as well as in theory.

My experience with the research grant system has, by and large, been pretty good. I cannot say the same thing for the contract system.

My personal experience with the contract system has led me to believe that it is wasteful and encourages duplicity. I am sure that it is not always this way, but I can only speak from my own experience.

The contract system has become the means by which second-rate scientists obtain first-rate financial support. This is not to say that people who have contracts are second-rate scientists. For some, it is their first experience with the contract system, and they have not yet found out what the drawbacks are—the drawbacks are never evident at the start. Some scientists may have so low an estimate of their own capacity to be judged in peer review that they would prefer the "sure thing" of a contract to possible rejection in the grant system. Some competent scientists are taking contract money because grant funds are just not available. There are also scientist-politicians who build their empires with contract money, and industries that are totally dependent on contract money for their existence. There are not very many independent scientists who, knowing both the grant and contract system, would choose the contract. The amount of red tape can be devastating, and the amount of busy-work a constant nuisance. In contrast, once a grant is obtained the scientist has almost complete freedom to pursue his interests, and the only thing that is required is an annual report each year during the period of the grant.

When a contract is put out to bid it is usually taken by someone. There is little possibility that, if there is no one to do the job who really knows what he is doing, that it will be dropped. Someone, somewhere, will move in to accept the bounty of the Cancer Institute.

Being basically a live and let live type of guy, I am somewhat reluctant to undercut a group of my fellow scientists who are working under the contract system. I would not do so unless I thought that it is necessary to abolish the contract system to keep from financially ruining creative cancer research. With the research grant system, the amount of money needed to do the research is related to the number of scientists performing it. In other words, you can expect the average scientist with his modest budget to consume a certain amount of money in supplies and assistance. He is limited by the amount of work that he can effectively control, and by how long it takes him to come up with a decent idea that seems to be worth pursuing. The contract system can continue to grow indefinitely. It follows Parkinson's law, so that eventually you can have a thousand people doing the work that was originally done by one. Since the people directing these programs have their hands on the purse strings, it will only be a matter of time before no one else can get into the act—which means the end of small independent projects. In short, the last bastion of individual thought in cancer research, while it would not be destroyed completely, would be seriously impaired by the preservation of the contract system.

Another danger of the contract system is that it tends to

place the control of research in the hands of a few people. The world is full of incompetents. While incompetence is a relative term, one thing is certain: *An incompetent man in a high position can do considerably more damage than he would do if he were in a lower position or in a small organization.* This argument will be countered by people who claim that an exceptionally competent individual in a position of power can do an immense amount of good. I believe that the danger of an incompetent getting into power considerably outweighs the benefit of an extremely competent man getting into power. It has been far more common to find incompetent megalomaniacs in positions of power than it has been to find exceptionally competent ones. Often highly intelligent and competent people prefer positions several rungs below the top. They are much more comfortable there, because they are not continually being sniped at.

A research contract uses private industry as an auxiliary arm of a government scientist to perform research. Most of the time—as is the nature of research—experiments are a complete bust. The answers that were sought are not obtained and the only return on the money spent is the information that the experiment, as tried, did not work. This is not unusual; it happens in all laboratories engaged in the business of research. There is a very important difference: The same research done in a university, even if it doesn't work, indirectly supports the training of embryo research scientists. If the experiment doesn't work, at least some student will learn a good deal from having performed it—and will know what not to do the next time. In an industrial setting, the same experiment can be repeated over and over and over again in the manner of the Sorcerer's Apprentice, without anybody learning anything. There is really no need to learn anything, because the more times you do the same experiment, the less the investment in learning and effort, and more money comes in.

I think that one of the reasons that the British have made such a disproportionately large number of discoveries is because their system tended to support the man rather than the work. By supporting the man, he is left free to follow his own curiosity wherever it may lead—and sometimes it leads to the proverbial pot of gold.

The nation as a whole, and the basic cause of cancer research (which is to understand what cancer is and to attempt to find remedies for it), would be served by the abolition of the entire research contract program. If the funds used for the contract program were funneled into the grants program, there would be enough money to finance a superb program of cancer research. As for the treatment of cancer patients, this would be best served by improving medical care in the nation as a whole; but it is not the purpose of this book to even suggest how this might be done.

Creative Federalism or Bureaucracy

The man who is a pessimist before forty-eight knows too much; the man who is an optimist after forty-eight knows too little.

Mark Twain

The intention of the planners of the National Cancer Institute were to make it a research center, and an administrative center for dispensing funds to various institutions around the country. From its inception, many scientists were afraid that the institute would grow so big and so powerful that it would control all of cancer research in the country. To prevent it from becoming a massive political structure exerting inordinate controls, its size was unofficially limited. There were no plans to guide the direction of cancer research in the country, only to encourage and finance it.

In the past a scientist who wished to solve a particular problem would present a proposal to the appropriate government agency. This proposal would be reviewed by a board of his peers (Study Section), and its suitability passed upon. He then received the money—or didn't. This is the essence of the "grant system," which is still very active. In recent years, the government has gravitated toward what they refer to as "creative federalism" in which a central planner describes what programs should be undertaken: The government says in essence, "We have a pile of money here to do such and such;

Who wants to do it?" The people who apply do so either because they are sincerely interested in the project, and would have done so anyway; or because they really want to do something else and this is a good way to get money to do it; or their company can use the money. This is the essence of the "contract system."

The government's philosophy has now changed, and more emphasis is being placed on large contract programs. This has been at the insistence of Congress. Many congressmen believe that things are moving too slowly. There has been a very powerful lobby that is pushing for a crash program to "cure cancer." In the last ten years or so a number of people have gained considerable influence in the cancer institute who believe that the institute should "direct" cancer research in the nation, and should decide in which direction research should go. These people have been becoming progressively more powerful to the point where they now control at least half the budget of the Cancer Institute. Are their plans of any value? I don't think so.

The volume of work and publication that has been generated from this new type of federal spending has been large— the quality of the work has been questionable. It is conceivable that under brilliant direction, this type of program can produce some exciting results. It is unlikely that more than one or two people with this type of ability could be found, and they would in no way be able to cover the number of programs that the government seems to be willing to sponsor. The result is, that there are perhaps a few good contract programs and many poor ones. In contrast to this, the research grant method tends to yield results in proportion to the total number of qualified and imaginative investigators.

Our experience has shown that poor workmanship can be tolerated only in something that can be thrown away. We tolerate all sorts of things in disposable knives, and forks and spoons. We can even tolerate shoddy buildings. In science, if the foundation is shoddy, the entire structure collapses. We need a firm fund of reliable information to build our theories and our understanding on. The type of research that is fostered by contracts has little room in it for quality control. When a man's personal reputation is at stake, he tends to be pretty careful about what he publishes—but when it can be cloaked in anonymity of a contract report, there is no telling what sins will be committed.

The government argument seems to be—"Look at the wonders that have been performed with things like industrial plastics, rocketry, and so forth. Why couldn't we do the same thing in cancer research?" The answer is fairly simple: If the background of information in cancer research was a fraction of the background of information in chemistry, electronics, and aerodynamics, perhaps we could.

When government support for institutions of higher education was proposed, there were many people who feared that this would mean control of these institutions by the government. There were all sorts of reassurances that this would not happen, but it has. It has happened because "Washington" controls the purse strings, and the man who pays the piper calls the tune. The government did not call the tune for a long time; it waited until the universities became dependent on government funds, and then it started. It is like Tom Lehrer's dope peddler who "gives the kids free samples, because he knows full well that today's young innocent faces will be tomorrow's clientele."

I used to classify myself as a "liberal" and a believer in government-run projects. I'm beginning to think, as Ambrose Bierce did, and as he defines this in *The Devil's Dictionary*, that the conservative is "A statesman who is enamored of existing evils, as distinguished from the Liberal, who wishes to replace them with others."

The Great Scientific Depression

The pundits say the jobless rate
Is what it ought to be.
But I resent that five percent,
'Cause part of THEM is ME.

At the 1968 meeting of the American Association for Cancer Research in Chicago, there was a man who was buttonholing everyone and asking if anyone knew where there was a job available. He brought back memories of that song of the great depression, "Brother, Can you Spare a Dime."

The heydays of fundamental research were the soaring '50s and '60s. Scientists in this country, and all over the world, were enthusiastic. The unprecedented financial support given to fundamental research was beginning to bear fruit. In all areas of cancer research, scientists were both busy and exuberant. The genetic code was being cracked; new and important discoveries were being made constantly in the field of cancer virus research; and exciting theories and experiments on how chemical carcinogens acted were being done; there was a possible chemical cure for acute leukemia, and choriocarcinoma had been cured chemically. In the quiet of their laboratories, scientists, who had started their work ten years before, were beginning to have their work bear fruit. For every discovery that made headlines, or excited the research community, there were others in the mill that were destined to do the same thing in the future.

The beginnings of the great scientific depression hit in 1968. Scientists were told that there was not enough money to finance the commitments made by the Cancer Institute (as well as other branches of the National Institutes of Health). Vast across-the-board cuts were made in every scientist's research budget. Many research grant renewals were not forthcoming, and the chances of applying and receiving a new grant were slim. Study sections began to apply their hatchet unmercifully.

How well I remember that 1968 meeting of the American Association for Cancer Research. It was like a wake. It was as if the whole cancer research apparatus was preparing to die. What happened in that year was a blow from which cancer research will not soon recover. Scientists, who were not particularly familiar with the intricacies of finance and politics, began to wonder what had happened. After many years of depending on government financing for cancer research, most people had come to expect that adequate support would continue indefinitely. Research programs that scientists thought were sound and should be continued were dropped, or their budgets substantially cut. How could the people in the National Cancer Institute and Congress have allowed this to happen? Scientists who had lost their support felt betrayed by the institute and the government—and for good reason.

In 1971 some hope appeared over the horizon. Congress had appropriated an additional one-hundred million dollars to add to the cancer research budget. At last, cancer scientists could go back to doing their research instead of starting to look for jobs in other areas. The joy was short-lived because it soon became evident that only a small amount of money—not enough to begin to revive independent cancer research—had been allocated to the grants and fellowship programs. Most of it was earmarked for large government projects. Scientists who wished to do as they were told could apply for contracts and, if they were obliging enough, would have little difficulty in getting one.

The independent scientist started looking around for a job with more of a future. When he looked outside of cancer research, he found that cancer research was not the only door being closed. Basic research in all areas was being curtailed, and university teachers were a dime a dozen.

It was fairly easy to predict what would happen with cancer research money should the times become leaner. It is much the same as what hapens to the remaining food supply in times of famine. In times of famine, those who are most ingenious in the production of food manage to retain enough food for themselves; while those who are able to con others out of food also manage to survive. This appears to be precisely what was happening in science. As the supply of research money dwindled, the remaining funds went to the potential Nobel Laureates, past Nobel Laureates, and the scientific con men. People in the middle were cut out, and the emerging young scientist stood little chance of being funded unless his doctoral thesis represented a major breakthrough—an unlikely possibility. When funds diminish, one might say that we support only geniuses and politicians.

No matter what is done financially, the creative scientist will not stop thinking. These national policies will not bring science grinding to a screeching halt, but they will divert many creative scientists from their laboratories to the production of contract applications, and to saving string. Being emotional human beings, some scientists who would ordinarily be thoughtful and careful workers may be prompted to publish for the sake of publishing—which is directly related to continued support. I know one who decided to write a popular book about cancer when his research money was cut off. We have no way of knowing what brand new discovery has been frustrated by these budget cuts any more than we know how many accidents may have been prevented by a "drive carefully" type of educational campaign.

I don't think that the public realizes how much of a disaster the Great Scientific Depression was and is. Scientists are very delicate instruments. They function best in a quiet secure atmosphere. A scientist thinks about science—which is about the most important thing that he does—unless he has to think about caring for his family and his future in general. When the depression hit me, the words of a wise friend of mine rang in my ears: Ten years ago, when I left a teaching position for one in which I would do nothing but research, he told me, "You're being foolish, Ira; what kind of a job is research? Teaching is a job; research is a hobby." I began to wish that I had taken his advice; because if I had, I would have been securely ensconced in a university, with tenure; my services as a teacher would be in demand, and I would not have been subject to the whims of the National Cancer Institute and Congress.

Who is to blame for the great depression? We can't blame the Republicans, because it was started under the Johnson administration. We can't blame the Democrats, because the subsequent Republican administration did nothing to correct the trend, but made it worse. We can't blame the National Cancer Institute because they were just following the instructions of Congress, and we can't blame Congress because they were doing what the National Cancer Institute told them was necessary. It was a case of "who killed Cock Robin?"

At the time of this writing, the Great Scientific Depression is in full swing. The national statistics haven't changed. There are no bread lines, and little perceptible unemployment, but it is here nevertheless. The public will never know how much damage has been done—what difference do a few productive years make in the life of a cancer research scientist, or on cancer research?

When a scientist cannot get the money to do the research that he feels should be done, he begins to look at that pie chart on how the money is distributed as if it were as a real pie. He thinks that the portion that he should have for his use is going to someone else, and tends to get a little paranoid. As Lewis Carroll put it—

> I passed by his garden, and marked, with one eye,
> How the Owl and the Panther were sharing a pie:
> The Panther took pie-crust, and gravy, and meat,
> While the Owl has the dish as its share of the treat.

When the pie was all finished, the Owl, as a boon,
Was kindly permitted to pocket the spoon:
While the Panther received knife and fork with a growl,
And concluded the banquet by ———

Lewis Carroll, *Alice's Adventures in Wonderland*

This reaction was typical among scientists who had either lost their research funds entirely or had them substantially reduced.

Before this depression hit, the attitude of the cancer research scientist was one of "live and let live." He thought, "What if the government does waste money on a drug screening program, or something else that will probably go nowhere; it's still supporting basic research. Besides, it's always possible that a boondoggle may produce something worthwhile." When he sees that his research funds are being cut, his work destroyed, and that his newly created scientists cannot get funds to do research nor even jobs, he begins to realize that the money for these boondoggles is not coming from nowhere, but is coming out of the budget that should rightfully be used for fundamental research. It has been slow in coming, but scientists are finally beginning to realize that there is a limit to the amount of money that is available for basic research, and that it will not be used for basic research if it is used for other programs. It is out of character for a scientist to sit still while his source of support is being whittled away. Many scientists are now beginning to howl.

Scientists, Research, and Discovery

The singer loves to sing. He asks society to allow him to do this. In exchange, he will make the sounds of the world more pleasant.

The scientist asks to be allowed to lift the skirts of the unknown. In exchange for this privilege, he might give many people some added years of life—or make their lives richer or more pleasant.

The key man in this business of cancer research is the scientist himself. There are many other people who are concerned with research, and if they are effective they keep the wheels turning smoothly. Administrators, technicians, and others can often make the difference between a job taking one year or ten years. But the key man in this enterprise is still the scientist—without him there is no enterprise. Harold L. Stewart has pointed out that there is little that scientists have in common. The only common element that characterizes all of them is a basic enthusiasm for what they are doing.

It is important to remember that a scientist is a scientist only when he is working at it. When he comes home, if he's a family man, he assumes the role of husband, father, repairer of broken toys, taxpayer, and the many other roles that every individual is called upon to play. Even in his job there may be times when his role is not that of a scientist. He may assume the role of teacher, administrator, committee member, architect.

I would like to make this point again because I think it is

important: The point is that a scientist is a scientist only when he is working at trying to solve a scientific problem. "Scientist" is an occupation like lawyer, plumber, or physician; it is not a title like "General" that follows a man to his grave. It is when "scientist" becomes a title that confusion arises. A man may start out as a scientist by receiving a Ph.D. (which is a title), work at being a scientist for a while, and then go into administration or into politics. While it is true that he is still capable of practicing the craft that he learned originally, this may not be what he is doing at all. If he realizes that what he is doing is administration or politics and not science, he can do his job reasonably well. If he is functioning in the administration or politics of science, then he knows enough to hire people who are actually engaged in doing science while he continues to perform his job.

The scientist may, in many ways, be in worse shape than the musician with regard to selling his products. The musician can point to a score, the artist to a painting, but the scientist's work—unless he is eminently successful—has no sale. In this sense, the picture of the creative scientist as a small man working in the corner of his laboratory, hoping that no one will notice him and take away his marbles, is not too far from wrong. This may be especially true of the exceptionally imaginative scientist who is far ahead of his time.

Fundamental research has no immediate utilitarian value. It comes out of the scientist as a work of art emerges from an artist. When his work becomes useful to the public, or popular as do works in the graphic arts or music, he will no longer have difficulty earning a living. But what does he do until that time comes? This poses no particular problem if, as the Prince of Monaco or the Emperor of Japan, he is born to the purple. If he is not independently wealthy, then there are several alternatives. He can work for a living and practice his art in his spare time. Universities offer this opportunity by paying a man to teach and allowing him the opportunity and the space to practice his art—which is research. Another alternative is to find a patron who will allow him to practice his art unimpeded by pecuniary considerations. But there are various kinds of patrons. The ideal patron is one who allows him to practice his art without interference. Such a patron might say to a composer, "Go and compose music. When you're done I'd like to hear it." For the scientist, such a patron was John D. Rockefeller and his institute, and the National Institutes of Health. There are other kinds of patrons. One type would hire a composer and tell him that "You can compose; but your compositions must be in the style of Beethoven." The dedicated creative artist will not be told how to practice his art, nor will the dedicated creative scientist. Failing to find a generous patron, he will probably turn to teaching for his livelihood, with research as his hobby. If he is a good teacher, then research's loss will be the teaching profession's gain. If he is a poor teacher, nobody gains. Some scientists, having little love for teaching, will accept the poor patron and turn out compositions in the style of Beethoven, while bootlegging their own art. Unfortunately, once corrupted, an artist has a slim chance of recapturing his integrity. He may even begin to enjoy the rewards that his hack work is producing, and will manage to convince himself that this work is real, and that his dreams are ethereal.

What is research, and why is it so unpredictable? Since scientists can put a man on the moon, why not a cure for cancer?

It is difficult to explain to a lay audience what the odds are of making an important scientific discovery. There are millions of people that have a pretty good idea of what the odds are of getting a golf ball into a hole with a single stroke; or two or three or four. There are relatively few who understand how small the probability is of making an important scientific discovery. But the probability is different for different scientists. The highly skilled, perceptive investigator is more likely to make a discovery than the duffer. Everyone has heard of the beginning golfer who makes a hole in one; and the equivalent happens (rarely) in science. To the professional golfer, the hole in one is also quite improbable, but a hole in two or three is very frequent. This is not true of the duffer.

One crucial variable, which makes research different

from golf, is that in research no one knows where the hole is. Therefore, the first problem is to find out where the hole is located; in other words, what is the problem that one has to solve? What some perceptive scientists do is to imagine the location of the hole (the problem) in their head and proceed to solve it. If you test it and the ball falls into the hole and the whole world cheers, you've done it. If the ball falls into the hole and no one cheers, you're never sure whether you've missed the boat (if I may mix metaphors) or have actually located the hole and sunk the ball, but the game isn't going to be played until next week.

There are as many different ways of doing research as there are of making music. Which way is correct? No one way is correct. All of the different approaches yield results of different kinds. All, in their own way, contribute to the advancement of our understanding. I should not say all, because some bits of research actually retard progress by cluttering up the literature with wrong information; which is considerably worse than no information at all.

Life styles in research are quite different. At one end of the spectrum is the scientist who directs a large operation involving many other scientists, massive numbers of technicians, large amounts of money, and virtually runs his own publishing house. At the other end of the spectrum is the individual who is working alone, sometimes with a little bit of technical help, who spends more time thinking than he does experimenting, and publishes only when he feels that he has truly solved a problem. There is a whole spectrum in between. Many scientists experiment with different life styles and do things in different ways at different times.

I've heard many creative scientists talk about doing two kinds of research: They say that they do *real* research and also have a "bread and butter" problem, which is the kind where you can see the end in sight and can therefore write a plausible project proposal in order to obtain money. You're also reasonably sure of a useful (?) publication at the end of the work. This "bread and butter" problem equips the laboratory, provides technicians, and so on. It also allows the scientist the time to do what most creative scientists consider to be the exciting stuff; the exploration of new and totally unpredictable frontiers. It allows him to do what Stewart calls "Sunday morning experiments," which are experiments that he's ashamed to do when anybody is watching. These are the long shot experiments which rarely pay off, but when they do, they pay off big.

The history of science is full of fortunate accidents falling upon the prepared mind. It is, in fact, the stuff that fine science is made of. Yet, for every one of these lucky accidents that turns out to be correct, there are thousands that end up in the waste basket, either because the observations are worthless, or because the tools to extract their meaning have not yet been discovered. The discovery by Gregor Mendel of the laws of heredity did not become truly meaningful until the role of the chromosomes was discovered. It was then that the brilliance of his observations became painfully evident. You can take ten scientists of equal ability and equal perceptiveness and, while all will produce work which is worthwhile, perhaps only one will make a startling discovery. It is much like walking through a maze. If the first turn that you take is wrong —and it is entirely accidental—someone else may have reached the goal ahead of you.

It would all be very nice if we could determine, in advance, who the creative scientists are going to be; and support them. There is no known way of doing this; any more than it is possible to determine from high school intelligence test scores, or grades, who is going to be the fine physician, architect, engineer, or war hero. We are forced to conclude that the man who is going to be successful is the one who becomes successful. It is necessary, therefore, to support a large number of scientists who will contribute relatively little in order to support the one who may contribute much. It is not too difficult for someone, who understands the field, to pick out a promising scientist once he has started to make good some of the promise. It is virtually impossible to do this at any earlier time. It is also impossible to predict when a previously productive scientist will stop being scientifically productive and will start cluttering the literature with his undocumented personal opinions as a few Nobel Laureates have done.

It is the very rare scientist who sets out to make a particular discovery and does it. Most discoveries are made by people who are trying to satisfy their curiosity about something, or by people who come upon something important by accident. More often than not, an individual goes into a particular branch of science because of some accident in his background (someone he loved died of cancer) or because some inspiring teacher "turned him on." Like that first critical turn in going through a maze, a good early choice is entirely accidental. The few people who have made outstanding discoveries in the process of performing the research for their doctoral thesis have done so because they were lucky enough to have a professor who pointed their nose in at least one fruitful direction. If not this, then it happened because they happened to be at a particularly good place at a particular time. This is not to say that brilliant people will not inevitably make some important discovery, but it might take them a considerably longer time; and they make it in an entirely different area. Pasteur did not set out to discover the cause of disease; he was interested in finding out what caused wine to sour. Jenner, the discoverer of smallpox vaccine, was perceptive enough to observe that milkmaids did not develop smallpox in the course of an epidemic, and associated the disease of cowpox with smallpox. Had he been in a different place, or in a different time, these fortuitous observations would not have been made. Even the well-known story of the discovery of the structure of DNA by Watson, Wilkins, and Crick could not have been made twenty years before the time it was made —even if the same people had gathered together at the same place. Freud did not set out to discover psychoanalysis. He would have been a biologist, but for the accident that he had to earn a living; and he did it as a physician. It is interesting that all of these men would probably have made significant scientific discoveries, but they would not have been the ones that they are now famous for.

The deliberate discovery of the physical structure of DNA was possible because there was already a reasonably large body of existing information. Besides the equipment for x-ray crystallography (no mean accomplishment in itself), there was the finding of Erwin Chargaff in 1949 that there were fixed proportions of adenine, thymine, guanine, and cytosine. These so-called base ratios made the discovery of the structure of DNA possible. Chargaff did not know where his discoveries would ultimately lead when he started to study the chemistry of DNA. Friedrich Meischer, who discovered DNA in 1896 in Germany, had the idea that DNA might be the genetic material. Meischer might not have fared so well in today's research funding climate in obtaining money for an apparently useless quest.

I think that it is safe to say that there are now scientists working on problems that no one else is interested in, whose findings will some day excite the scientific world. It is also safe to say that there are scientific findings already published that no one is paying very much attention to, which will also someday excite the scientific community when it is ready for them.

A number of articles have pointed out that the public is impatient with the amount of time that scientists are taking. An excellent article on "The Politics of Cancer" concludes with a statement that "It [the congressional battle about financing cancer research] should make clear to the public, on one hand, that it cannot expect instant cures to cancer—and that Congress anyway cannot legislate the remedies. On the other hand, it should serve as ample reminder to scientists that the public has a deep stake in their research, and that it will not tolerate for too long the ivory tower attitudes that sometimes do creep into their work. The scientists will have to give a convincing performance that they are, indeed, progressing toward practical payoffs." * Attitudes like this, which insist on evidence of practical payoffs or convincing performance, will have the same effect on cancer research as telling the doctor who is trying to remove something from your eye to "Stop diddling around, and get the damn thing out."

* Russell, Christine, "The Politics of Cancer," *The Washington Post,* November 28, 1971.

How Goes the War Against Cancer?

Our greatest pretenses are built up not to hide the evil and the ugly in us, but our emptiness. The hardest thing to hide is something that is not there.

Eric Hoffer, *The Passionate State of Mind*

The people who are concerned about cancer (at least those who are presently influential) have apparently decided that, since the Pentagon is the only branch of government that consistently gets all of the money that it asks for, they should adopt Pentagon strategy. They have not only declared "War On Cancer," but have adopted the entire lexicon of Pentagonese to fight the war with. It is probably a tactical error since (I think) the American public has had a bellyfull of war. We now have cancer task forces,* and the war against cancer has even acquired its own fort. Fort Deitrich, once the bastion of the chemical and biological warfare programs, is now part of the "War Against Cancer." If there is a "War Against Cancer" —well—how goes the war?

"The War against Cancer is being waged against unbelievably difficult odds. Considerable progress has been made on all fronts, but it is still a hard uphill fight." Translated from military language, this means that those of us who are

* Russell Baker defines task force as "any group appointed by the President's advisory program for Congress to ignore." Russell Baker, "The Vast Wasteland of Hard Nosed Multi-gigaton Words, *New York Times*, September 17, 1961.

fighting the war against cancer are getting the s _ _ t kicked out of us. Lung cancer, due to smoking, continues to climb; and while the leukemia rate appears to be decreasing, it is still at least twice what it was in 1923. Even if the most extravagant claims of the cancer therapists are true, and they are actually curing the number that they say they are, it is still a drop in the bucket compared to the number of new cases. If the 160 cures for leukemia (assuming that they are really cures) are equated against the number of new cases that have come into being in the last year (19,000), the overview is pathetic. Deaths due to cancer of the uterine cervix have been steadily decreasing. This is probably due to the increased use of the Pap smear, and the removal of tumors of the uterus long before they have begun to spread. There has been one notable victory: cancer of the stomach has dropped precipitously to unprecedented levels—but we don't have the faintest idea how we did it. If a business were doing as poorly as the "War Against Cancer," there would be an immediate outcry by the stockholders for a complete change in top management. One thing is certain: the business of dealing with the cancer problem is too important to declare bankruptcy.

Is the time ripe for a crash program to either discover the cause or the cure for cancer? Let us deal with both of these separately:

With regard to the cause of cancer, I would like to refer you back to Part II on "What We Don't Know About Cancer." There are large, essential pieces of information about cancer that are still missing. Even if there were not big pieces missing, finding the "cause" of something does not ordinarily yield to crash programs. It is solving technologic problems that succumbs to an all-out effort.

People who think that the time is right for a crash program to find a cure point to the chemical cure of choriocarcinoma, and the improved treatment, and possible cure, of acute leukemia. The results of the treatment of these two diseases is very encouraging. It is so much better than anything that has ever existed, that it is not surprising that it generates considerable enthusiasm. There is also no question that a con-

siderable effort should be devoted to perfecting the treatment
of acute leukemia and choriocarcinoma. At the present time
a fraction of the patients who could be cured are treated. The
treatment that works with choriocarcinoma and acute leukemia
has proved to be ineffective with other forms of cancer, even
those closely related to them. Therapists claim that these new
treatments should be made available to all people with these
two forms of cancer. I agree with this completely—this could
be done by the general improvement of our medical facilities.
The idea that you could have a ramshackle hospital, with an
inefficient, poorly trained staff, and a superb cancer chemotherapy unit with a superbly trained cancer chemotherapist,
is nonsense. In order to attack cancer (not just the few forms
that yield to chemotherapy) a fine general hospital is needed.
It is needed because the first important stage in handling
cancer is diagnosis, which requires good departments of pathology, internal medicine, and gynecology. It needs a good department of surgery to treat most forms of cancer; and at the
end of the line, we need a chemotherapy department to treat
the cases that will yield to chemotherapy, and to palliate
others. When this is all organized, you no longer have a
"Cancer Center," but you have built a "Medical Center." In
terms of meeting this total need, the amounts of money currently proposed for cancer programs would be a drop in the
bucket. What is now being proposed sounds a bit like building
a two bedroom house with ten baths.

Advocates of contract research point to some of the successes in chemotherapy, and attribute them to the Cancer
Chemotherapy Program, the prototype for contract research
programs. While this program provided much of the money
to perfect chemotherapy, it was not responsible for the discoveries that led to effective treatments. Most of the important
discoveries in chemotherapy were not made by the random
screening of chemicals—the major part of the contract
program.

I would like to make it clear that I think that chemotherapy research has been important, is important now, and
will be important in the future. Like any other form of re-

search, the value received by the public will be proportional to the ability of the people doing the research. Research in chemotherapy needs the same perceptiveness, intelligence, judgment, and all of the other things needed for good science. The best in chemotherapeutic research has been done by people who knew how to carefully control experiments, had a good fundamental knowledge of chemistry and experimental biology, and abiding interest in what makes things grow.

One of the objectives of the Cancer Chemotherapy screening program was to screen large numbers of chemicals for their anticancer activity. It is likely, from what I have seen of the program, that much time was spent on chemicals that were either ineffective, or were too toxic to have any value; and that some potentially effective substances were screened by the methods used and discarded. The Cancer Chemotherapy Program was heavily funded by Congress and the result was that large numbers of chemicals were screened at considerable cost. I believe that the useful findings of the chemotherapy program could have made at considerably less expense had the research been funded through the research grants system. Furthermore, had the same amount of money been put into the grant system, we might know much more about how tumors behave than we do now. What I have just said is my personal opinion, and it would be impossible to document it objectively. I have been singularly unimpressed with the management of the Cancer Chemotherapy Program, and believe that the nation's interest would be best served by eliminating it. I also believe that this opinion is shared by many of the most competent cancer scientists in the country. It is probably not shared by people that are presently receiving the largest amount of their financial support from the Cancer Chemotherapy Program. The competent investigators should have little difficulty receiving equivalent support for the same work via the grant system—provided that the money is available.

The government very recently decided that one of the promising areas in cancer research is cancer immunology and cancer virology. Money is available, in research contracts, to study these areas, and research institutes all over the country are beginning to advertise for qualified applicants. First, the total number of immunologists and virologists is a relatively small number. Of these, the ones that are skilled in the cancer end of their fields is a still smaller part of this group. Of these skilled cancer virologists and immunologists, most are already productively employed in universities, medical schools, research institutes, and so forth. With enough money, perhaps some could be induced to leave—but it should be pointed out that every time a scientist changes his location, his work is set back by a substantial period of time (I estimate at least two years for me). The effect of suddenly putting money into the immunology and virology programs will not be to accelerate research in this area, but to retard it.

The argument will be advanced that more scientists would develop an interest if the financial rewards were made available. This is probably not true; a scientist's interests are determined by very many factors, the least of which is money. There has been a crying need for people to teach human gross anatomy in medical schools. This has not led to an increase in the number of gross anatomists; on the contrary, the number is continually going down. The reason that it is going down is because the field is, for many reasons, basically unattractive to many who would ordinarily be qualified to pursue it. If there are a limited number of qualified and dedicated cancer immunologists in the country, increasing the number of jobs available for cancer immunologists is not going to add more qualified, enthusiastic immunologists. It might conceivably encourage cancer immunologists to train more people in this field —but who knows what the fad is going to be in ten or twenty years, when these new scientists hit the job market. In short, science by fad is doomed to failure.

What Can and Can't Be Done—
An Editorial

Grant me the serenity to accept the things I cannot change;
courage to change the things I can; and wisdom to know the
difference.

Francis of Assisi

If I were asked to suggest a science policy which the government could follow, I would have to distinguish very clearly
between the basic and the applied sciences.

For the support of basic research, I think that imaginative
people should be supported, and that their work should be
supported without taking into consideration any possible practical applications of that work. If a scientist appears to have
talent, his work should be supported, with no one telling him
what to do or how to do it. This system worked quite well in
the Kaiser Wilhelm Institute in pre-World War II Germany,
where they managed to collect the greatest array of scientific
brain power that the world had seen up to that time. The
Rockefeller Institute operated on the same premise—and very
successfully. The National Institutes of Health, by and large,
operated on that basis, despite the fact that on the surface
it appeared to support projects rather than individuals. Their
attitudes appear to be changing.

My major objection to what is happening in cancer research is that research, once the province of the individualist,
the independent spirit, the free thinker, is now being taken

over lock, stock, and barrel by the same type of bureaucracy that operates the military, and the space program. Where can a scientist who wishes to retain his independence and freedom go? His patron, the government, has not only let him down, but is now in the business of trying to persuade him to sell himself, body and soul, to a "higher authority."

I went into research because I never did like being told what to do—it makes little difference to me whether I am being told what to do by a Lieutenant in the army, a Government Official, a Senator, or the President—I still don't like it. A colleague of mine recently told me that I didn't have to sell my soul—just make a few compromises with the government. I didn't tell him this, but making compromises with power *is* selling my soul. I can compromise with individuals, but not with the state.

A basic scientist wants nothing more than to be able to follow his nose. He is also human, and likes to live reasonably well—although not necessarily opulently. I would like to point out that such a policy, of supporting scientists without directing them, can bring incalculable benefits to society. The scientist is the explorer of the future. Explorers can open up vast new territories for exploitation. Basic research is also relatively inexpensive, when compared to applied research.

I talked to a professional politician whose attitude was "We know that scientists are only trying to feather their own nests, and don't have anything real to offer." He may be correct, with regard to the "scientists" he meets in Washington. He is also right about scientists wanting most of the things that anyone else wants. Yet, I have met relatively few greedy people outside the administrative structures of large organizations. The scientists who do the work are not greedy people. Most of the people who deliver your mail, teach your children, write your newspapers are not excessively greedy. They want their share—their small corner of the world. Most are satisfied if they are allowed to raise a family, and to live and die with a certain amount of dignity.

To be effective, any program that has as its goal either research or therapy has to have, as its first priority, the people who will do the work. A program that does not do this is doomed to failure. *The great mistake of the current cancer program is in placing people at the bottom of the priority ladder and programs at the top*—rather than the other way around.

It is obvious that the president, not being a cancer expert, cannot effectively determine policy with regard to cancer research and treatment. Neither can Congress nor the administrative structure of the National Cancer Institute. Yet, the president and Congress are responsible for the legislation which supports cancer research and treatment, and the administrative structure of the National Cancer Institute is charged with the responsibility for its execution. What is needed is a separate body which recommends policy to the president and Congress. This was the purpose of the National Advisory Cancer Council. The council still exists, but it now also has a troika which recommends directly to the president. The effectiveness of this arrangement will be a function of the ability and understanding of the men occupying these key positions. Unfortunately, most people who reach such positions of power have vested interests in the form of cancer institutes, universities, medical schools, or industry. Some may have fanatical commitments to pet ideas. It is hard to find competent people who do not have some vested interest of one form or another. It is, therefore, important to maintain representation for a wide number of interests, and a good deal of external surveillance in an attempt to insure that the members of these groups do not feather their own nests at the expense of the public interest. At the same time, it is important that this surveillance not be so great as to squelch all possibilities of creativity and innovation. This is the basic dilemma in any form of representative government. To make things more difficult, even honest and good men are often corrupted by power.

High-level bureaucrats are people that administer. They do not, as a rule, initiate programs. The attitude of the professional civil servant is very evident in the book by Dean Acheson, the former Secretary of State, entitled *Present at the Creation*. Nowhere in the book is there a hint that he was concerned about where national policy was leading, and how it was arrived at. His sole concern was the way in which it was executed. It is this type of monomania that drives people to the top of the bureaucratic ladder. It is as if even a whisper of disagreement with what Congress or the president decreed would cause a professional bureaucrat to be struck by a bolt of lightning (bureaucrats who attempted to make policy have been crucified in the past). Given a job to do, a top-level bureaucrat will get it done. It is this type of dedication that was responsible for most governmental accomplishments. It was also responsible for such monuments to idiocy as The Pyramids, The Charge of the Light Brigade, and others too numerous to mention. Perhaps that is the way it has to be. For a top-level bureaucrat to question the wisdom of the president and Congress would be analogous to a mailman questioning whether the delivery of junk mail was really worth his time. One should, therefore, never expect a bureaucrat to decide whether or not something is worth doing. There have, of course, been exceptions—people who have headed government bureaus who were able to advise Congress and the president as to policy. It is those people who advise the president and Congress who determine policy. Whether or not the policy is implemented is a function of public opinion and the effectiveness of lobbies. The fact that medical research is supported at all is largely an accomplishment of the "cancer lobby." In other areas of public policy, public opinion is influenced principally by the press (including radio and TV). The "science and medicine" press is not effective as an instrument of public opinion since its readers are largely members of the professions. Lobbies, therefore, have an inordinately large influence. The drive of the cancer lobby was counterbalanced by several powerful spokesmen for the relatively conservative scientific establishment. At the present time, the scientific representatives appear to have been "hand picked" by the lobby itself. With everyone agreeing that a crash program is the thing to have and that directed research is the way to solve the cancer problem, it is not surprising that that is the way things are being done. The scientific community does not appear to have an effective spokesman who understands science as well as politics. Policy with regard to cancer research is now being determined by people who are not scientists nor medical practitioners. They, in turn, are being inordinately influenced by a handful of scientist-politicians who are imbued with the same evangelistic zeal as their mentors. They have managed to lose sight of reality and have converted cancer research into a giant political game. For them, the fight against cancer is not fought in the hospitals and laboratories, but in the newspapers and magazines.

I would like to give as the reason for the support of fundamental research an impressive record of accomplishment. Compared to what remains to be done, what we have accomplished so far does not seem impressive, yet, compared to what has been accomplished in other areas, and in the past, it is pretty impressive: After all, what can any group of people accomplish in a lifetime? Congress and the president have given us a government that has a remarkable capacity for spending a lot of money for relatively little. Government has created massive amounts of red tape; but in its favor, the nation is still intact and functioning. Physics has given us the atom bomb and nuclear power; chemistry has given us better things for better living; and the military has apparently solved the problem of being able to keep a nation at war forever without actually winning it or losing it. The alliance of basic biological research with the medical scientist has given us penicillin and a wide variety of other antibiotics, the potential for eradicating a number of diseases, and above all, is informing the public that we may be destroying ourselves and should do something to stop it. We can prevent a variety of deadly diseases such as smallpox, bubonic plague, diphtheria —to name just a few. We now understand much about how we are put together, both chemically and physically. There are so many things which we now take for granted that were not even in existence one hundred years ago—we even know how to prevent lung cancer, as well as how to cause it.

There are many things that the government can spend money for in order to keep the wheels of the economy turning, and I can think of nothing better to pour it into than basic biological research. It primes the economy in the same way that military spending does. Research employs people, engenders the production of new goods, and keeps creative people doing constructive things such as scientific experiments—instead of writing muckraking books. Basic research can potentially enhance the lives of everyone, even though there is no clear-cut timetable. The same rationale might also be given for the support of elementary education, art, music, intellectual history, and a wide variety of other human intellectual pursuits —enough support to keep the stewpots of the world filled. Basic research is a far better pastime for men than the invention of new and better ways to kill one another.

We have to keep up the research that will yield the tools of the future. This has to be done, not tomorrow, but now; because the years that a talented scientist does not spend doing research will never be recaptured. Talent has to be fostered, encouraged, nurtured—not tomorrow, but now. The time that has been lost due to cuts in research budgets in the last five years will never be retrieved. It does little good to talk about crash programs for the future when there are programs that are already in existence that are important and sound that need financial support.

In the area of applied science, a good deal remains to be done with tools now available. The statements now being made in the press by people in authority are leading the public to believe that cancer cannot be cured today. They are ignoring the many things that can be done, not tomorrow—but right now. Many cancers are curable by methods available today if they are only treated in time. We could, with constructive political leadership, prevent over 90 percent of cases of lung cancer, and it is conceivable that we might be able to reduce the incidence of leukemia by half. This is not with any new discovery or any wonderful tool of the future—this is with the knowledge that we have available today. This emphasis on a new chemical cure in the future is hampering the perfection of the tools that we have available now. The treatment of breast cancer by surgery needs detailed analysis and perfection so that the surgery can be made less debilitating. There appear to have been substantial inroads made in mortality due to cancer of the uterus by the simple use of the Pap smear. It is high time that we tested methods of detection for breast cancer and cancer of the lower bowel. They may be of no avail, or may be very effective in reducing deaths due to these cancers. We will have no way of knowing until they have been adequately tested. The time to try is now!

The government is far from willing to give financial carte blanche to cancer research. This is not likely to happen, since financial carte blanche is an extremely wasteful way of proceeding, and (advocates of the War Against Cancer notwithstanding) there are many equally important things that have to be done in the country and in the world. It is important, therefore, to make the best possible use of the money that is available for cancer research.

In dealing with the "applied" problem of cancer, there are some things which clearly can be accomplished. These are—

1. Humane treatment can be given to people suffering from both curable and incurable forms of cancer. This will go along with improving the overall quality of medical care in the nation.

2. A good many cases of cancer can be prevented—i.e., most cases of lung cancer could be prevented if people did not smoke cigarettes; radiation-induced cancer can be prevented by reducing the amount of radiation in our environment.

3. Programs of an educational and medical nature can be designed which increase early detection and early treatment of cancer.

4. Support can be provided for research on methods of detection and treatment.

Among the things that cannot be accomplished are the following:

1. A crash program which will cure cancer in 5 years, 10 years, 50 years, or 1,000 years for that matter. There is no way at the present time of predicting the outcome of existing research. I understand the need to be practical. If the government decided to use every bit of "cancer money" in a crash

program to eliminate cigarette smoking, and with it lung cancer; and to drastically reduce the amount of environmental radiation which might well halve leukemia incidence and reduce environmental pollution to eliminate a variety of potential cancer-causing agents, I would consider it to be a reasonable decision. But to spend one-third of the cancer budget on a crash program to find a "cure" at this stage of the game is, when compared to other needs, ill advised.

2. Production of a vaccine to prevent cancer.

3. A program designed to bring the benefits of medical science (whatever that is) to the public in the area of cancer or heart disease, or stroke—as something separate from improving the general quality of medical care in the nation.

I have made a distinction between what I believe can be done and cannot be done. Whether you agree with the wisdom of this distinction may in the large measure determine what is done in this country about the cancer problem.

A Cancer Glossary

ADENOCARCINOMA   A cancer of gland cells.

ADENOMA   A tumor of gland cells—usually benign.

ANAPLASTIC   An adjective that implies a reversion to a primitive state. Used to describe a relative lack of organized microscopic structure in the tumor.

ANDROGEN   A male sex hormone.

ANGIOMA   A tumor of blood or lymph vessels (hemangioma, a tumor of blood vessels; and lymphangioma, a tumor of lymph vessels).

ATROPHY   Diminution in size (the opposite of hypertrophy).

BENIGN   A tumor or condition that is not likely to kill.

BIOPSY   Taking out a small part of a tumor in order to find out what type it is.

BLAST   The immature form of blood cells of all types.

BRONCHOGENIC CARCINOMA   The most common form of lung cancer in man; it is composed of cells which look more like skin than they do the normal lining of the lung.

CANCER   Read the rest of the book!

CARCINOGEN   A cancer-producing substance.

CARCINOMA   A cancer made up of epithelial cells (as opposed to connective tissue cells).

CHEMOTHERAPY   The treatment of disease or tumors with the use of chemicals.

CHRONIC   Continuing for a long time—a condition that neither lets you get better nor die—as opposed to acute, which either kills you quickly or gets better quickly.

CIRCUMCISION   Removal of the foreskin of the penis.

COMPETENCE   The ability of an organ or part to perform adequately any function required of it—in people, this usually refers to the functioning of the brain (see *The Peter Principle* by Laurence Peter and Raymond Hull for a definition of incompetence).

CONNECTIVE TISSUE   The tissues that hold together everything else. Scars are made of connective tissue, as is most of the skin. Leather was once connective tissue.

CURE   The act of being made well—until you die. In cancer treatment, the usual criterion is survival for five or more years following the end of treatment, without sign of the tumor.

CYST   A hollow sac containing liquid or semisolid substance; may be mistaken for a true tumor.

DEATH   The inevitable consequence of life.

DIAGNOSIS   1. The art of distinguishing one disease from another. 2. Giving a name to the disease that you have, so that you can tell your friends about it.

DIET   (Gr. *diaita* way of living) The alteration of one's eating habits as a remedy for almost any disease but obesity.

DISEASE   What people have that makes them not feel well. This term should only be applied to people that have been seen by a physician and so pronounced.

DRUG   A chemical compound capable of curing or killing or neither.

EPIDERMIS   The outer layer of the skin.

EPITHELIOMA   A cancer of epithelial cells. The person originally classifying it could not make up his mind whether it was a cancer (in which case it would be called a carcinoma) or not.

EPITHELIUM   The covering of the internal and external surfaces of the body and cells derived from them. Everything that isn't connective tissue (connective tissue is everything that isn't epithelium). It includes the cells that comprise most of the skin, lungs, intestine, liver, kidney, and so on.

ESTROGEN   A female sex hormone of the type that produces "heat" in animals.

ETIOLOGY   A word that implies that the writer thinks that he understands what is causing something (e.g., the viral etiology of cancer).

EXAMINATION   To look at—and occasionally to see something.

EXPERIMENT   What scientists do at work; as distinguished from "trial" which is what therapists do at work.

EXTIRPATE   To take out, or to destroy utterly.

FIBROADENOMA   A benign tumor containing both glandular and connective tissues.

FIBROMA   A benign tumor composed of connective tissue.

GASTRIC   Pertaining to the stomach.

GASTRIC CARCINOMA   Cancer of the stomach.

GLAND   An organ that secretes, such as a sweat gland, salivary gland, or one that secretes hormones. Mammary gland is another name for breast.

GONAD   The ovary or the testis.

GRANULOCYTE   A type of white blood cell formed in the bone marrow and containing identifiable granules.

GRANULOMA   A benign tumor of connective tissue; usually occurring in response to irritation, infection, or the presence of a foreign body.

HEMANGIOMA   A benign tumor made up of blood vessels.

HEMANGIOSARCOMA   A malignant tumor made up of blood vessels.

HEMATO   A prefix meaning pertaining to blood.

HEMATOLOGIST   A specialist in diseases of the blood and blood-forming tissues.

HEMOGLOBIN   The red pigment of the blood.

HEMORRHAGE   A lot of bleeding.

HEMORRHOIDS   Piles; a blood vessel enlargement around the anus. If you've got them, you know what they are.

"HERPES SIMPLEX"   Cold sores (or the virus that causes them).

HISTOLOGY   Microscopic anatomy.

HODGKIN'S DISEASE   (Thomas Hodgkin, English physician, 1798–1866). A tumor of the cells involved in chronic infection. This was originally thought to be a form of tuberculosis, which it is not. It is a malignant tumor with a very variable growth rate; so that people sometimes survive for as much as thirty years with it. It is treatable with chemicals and x-ray, and may be completely curable.

HORMONE   A substance secreted by one organ (usually an endocrine gland) which exerts its effects on another organ.

HOSPITAL   An institution where sick people sometimes get well and well people sometimes get sick.

HYPERPLASIA   An abnormal increase in the number of cells; a "tumor" always involves hyperplasia.

HYPERTROPHY   The increase in the size of an organ. This can be due to hyperplasia, or it can be due to the increase in the size of the individual cells—as occurs in the enlargement of the muscles as a consequence of exercise.

HYPOPLASIA   The opposite of hyperplasia—decrease in cell number.

HYPOTHESIS   Where a scientist says he is going to go—often after he has gotten there.

HYSTERECTOMY   The removal of the uterus—a good way of getting rid of tumors of it.

IATROGENIC DISEASE   Diseases that are produced by the physician.

IMMUNOLOGY   The science which concerns itself with the defense system of an animal.

INCISION   A cut made by a surgeon.

INFLAMMATION   The response of the body to injury. It can be brought about by a direct injury, a foreign body, or an infection. The process is similar in all cases, and involves reddening of the area, heat, and usually pain.

INTESTINE   The medical term for gut.

KELOID   Excessive growth of skin in response to injury with an excessive amount of scar tissue.

LESION   An injury of any kind—whether it hurts or not.

LEUKEMIA   (White blood) A cancer of the blood forming cells.

LEUKOCYTE   A white blood cell (as distinguished from erythrocyte, which is a red blood cell).

LEUKOPLAKIA   White thickened patches on the inside of the

cheek and tongue. Believed to be precancerous. It is associated with smoking.

LIFE   See death.

LIVER   In France, the seat of the soul.

LYMPHOCYTE   White blood cell which inhabits both the blood and the lymph nodes. It is involved in immunity and chronic infection. Cancers of this cell are referred to as lymphocytic (or lymphatic) leukemia, or lymphosarcoma.

LYMPHOCYTOSIS   An increase in the number of circulating lymphocytes in the blood. This can be caused by many virus infections, and chronic infections in general, as well as by lymphocytic tumors.

MACROPHAGES   Large cells of the defense system of the body which eat bacteria and other foreign substances.

MALIGNANT   Tending to get worse. A malignant disease or a malignant tumor is one that is potentially lethal.

MAMMARY   Pertaining to the breast—comes from the word *mamma.*

MARROW, BONE MARROW   The soft material that fills up the cavities of the bones. Most blood cells, both red and white, are manufactured there.

MASTECTOMY   The surgical removal of the breast.

MASTITIS   Inflammation of the breast—a fairly common occurence which often frightens women into thinking that they might have cancer of the breast. Worth checking up on.

MEDICINE   1. Any drug or remedy. 2. The art that physicians practice—but rarely perfect.

MELANOMA   A tumor of the pigment cells of the body, usually black in color.

METASTASIS   The spread of tumors to distant parts of the body, and their establishment there.

METHODOLOGY   A word frequently used by scientists and government officials when they mean "method."

MICRO   A prefix meaning extremely small.

MITOSIS   A fancy word for one cell dividing into two in the usual way. Sometimes distinguished from meiosis which is cell division that takes place in the gonads in a somewhat different way (that is usual for the gonad).

MONOCYTE A large white blood cell found in the blood, which would be called a macrophage if it were found anywhere else in the body.

MONONUCLEOSIS (Infectious Mononucleosis) A viral disease, often spread by kissing, which results in the presence of large numbers of white blood cells in the blood. An unskilled observer might confuse this with leukemia. It is usually a self-limiting disease with only occasional complications.

MORTALITY The quality of being alive.

MOUSE A rodent that is to cancer research what the hammer is to the carpenter.

MYELOCYTE The primitive bone marrow cell that gives rise to the granulocyte.

MYELOID Pertaining to the cells produced by the bone marrow.

MYELOMA A tumor found in the bone marrow. Multiple myeloma is a tumor of plasma cells (see plasmacytoma) that metastasizes regularly to the bone marrow—hence its name.

MYOMA A tumor made up of muscle cells.

NEOPLASM A tumor.

NEOPLASTIC CHANGE Going from a "normal" to a "tumorous" stage.

NEURINOMA (Neuroma) A benign tumor of a nerve.

NEUROFIBROMA A tumor of the connective tissue of the nerve or of the nerve sheath.

NEUROFIBROMATOSIS Also called von Recklinghausen's disease. A condition inherited as a Mendelian dominant which predisposes its bearer to the development of a variety of conditions, the most consistent of which is the presence of neurofibromas.

NEUROGENIC SARCOMA A cancer of the connective tissue of the nerve.

NORMAL What you and I are, as distinguished from what other people are.

OESTRUS (Estrus) In sexual heat (Oelephants in oestrus are sometimes incoestrus).

ONCOLOGY The study of tumors.

ONCOLYTIC Anything that destroys tumor cells.

ONCOLOGIST   One who studies tumors—that's what I am.

OPERATION   Cutting into it or cutting it out.

OSTEOMA   A tumor of bone tissue.

PALPABLE   Can be felt with the hand.

PAPILLOMA   A wartlike tumor.

PATHOGNOMONIC   Specifically distinctive or characteristic of a disease or pathologic condition. A word which should never have been invented—when a book says that such and such a symptom is pathognomonic of such and such a disease, it probably isn't.

PATHOLOGY   (Also called morbid anatomy) The branch of medicine that treats of the essential nature of disease.

PATHOLOGISTS   Are generally concerned with the diagnosis of tumors, the laboratory diagnosis of disease, and post-mortem diagnosis. They always have the last word.

PHAGOCYTE   Cells that eat microorganisms or foreign bodies —granulocytes and macrophages are phagocytes.

PH. D.   Doctor of Philosophy; people can receive Ph.D. degrees in chemistry, zoology, anatomy, biochemistry, and a wide variety of other scientific disciplines. It is even possible to get a Ph.D. in philosophy.

PHYSICIAN   An authorized practitioner of medicine—As distinguished from those that are not authorized.

PLACEBO   (L. I will please) A substance of no medicinal value (sugar, and so on) given to a patient to make him feel better, or as a control in a therapeutic trial. They are often quite effective in making people feel better.

PLASMACYTOMA   (Also called multiple myeloma or myeloma) A tumor composed of plasma cells—the cells that make antibodies. This tumor metastasizes regularly to the bone marrow.

PLASMA CELL   The cell that manufactures antibodies.

PNEUMONECTOMY   The removal of a portion of the lung.

PNEUMONIA   An inflammation of the lungs. A common form is caused by a bacteria and is curable with antibiotics. Another form caused by a virus is curable by rest and prayer.

POLYP   A protruding tumor, usually of the digestive tract or upper respiratory tract.

POLYPOSIS A condition characterized by a number of intestinal polyps. The tendency to develop numerous intestinal polyps can be inherited.

PRECANCEROUS A condition which occurs before the development of a cancer. For example, leukoplakia of the mouth is a precancerous lesion, predisposing one to cancer of the cheek or tongue.

PROCTOSCOPE A super-duper-pooper-snooper's peeper.

PROSTATE A gland in the male located at the neck of the bladder. It secretes part of the normal ejaculate. It sometimes increases in size in older men, causing difficulty in urination; and sometimes becomes cancerous.

PROSTATECTOMY An operation which removes the prostate.

QUACK (A derogatory designation) 1. Someone who practices medicine without a license to do so. 2. A licensed physician who practices medicine dishonestly or dangerously. Cancer quacks can be either.

RADICAL Directed to the cause.

RADICAL SURGERY Surgery directed to the cause; such as amputation of the head to cure a headache.

RADIOLOGY The branch of medicine which deals with the use of ionizing radiation in the diagnosis and treatment of disease.

RADIOTHERAPY The treatment of disease using ionizing radiation.

RADIUM A radioactive element which emits ionizing radiation and is used in the treatment of cancer.

RECTUM The last five inches of intestine—ending at the anus.

REMISSION Relief from the symptoms of a disease. Usually used in reference to a disease which is not cured and is expected to recur. A spontaneous remission is one that is unrelated to any treatment.

RETICULOENDOTHELIAL SYSTEM The defense system of the body. This was originally used to refer to the system of phagocytic (eating) cells but has since been extended to include most of the elements of the defense system in-

cluding the antibody forming cells (no matter what definition I give to this term, someone is going to disagree).

RIGIDITY   Stiffness or inflexibility, chiefly that which is abnormal or morbid—a common characteristic of most older
members of most professions.

ROENTGENOLOGY   Synonymous with radiology.

ROENTGENOTHERAPY   Synonymous with radiation therapy.

SARCOID   Resembles a sarcoma, but is generally due to some
inflammatory process. It is not generally malignant.

SARCOMA   A cancer of the connective tissue, muscle, bone,
fat, the reticuloendothelial system, and so on—everything
but epithelium.

SCIENCE   That accumulated body of systematized knowledge
which has been obtained by scientists, Christian scientists,
physicians, dentists, historians, philosophers, healers of all
sorts, writers, brewmasters, bootleggers, mafiosi.

SCIENTIST   One who practices science.

SCROTUM   The sac that contains the testicles.

SICK   In American, meaning not in good health. In some parts
of England, a person who is only slightly under the weather
is "queer," one who is in serious condition is "ill" and one
who is menstruating is "sick." (Men never get sick in
England.)

SIGN   An indication of the existence of something—such as
that a doctor practices here. Babinski's sign indicates that
Dr. Babinski practices here. (That sign usually says Babinski and Kernig, M.D.)

SKIN   That part of an animal that comes off when he is
skinned—in man it consists of an epithelial layer (epidermis) and a connective tissue layer (dermis).

S.O.B.   Shortness of breath.

SUTURE   To sew; the thread used to sew with.

SYMPTOM   A clue to the nature of the disease.

SYNDROME   A set of symptoms which occur together and
distinguish a single disease. Syndromes usually have someone's name attached because the symptoms are too long to
list in one title, e.g., Gerstmann's syndrome: a combination

of finger agnosia, right-left disorientation, agraphia, acalculia, right homonymous diplopia and, in addition, right homonymous hemaniopsia, due to left-sided lesion in the angular gyrus—see what I mean!

TESTIS   (testicle) The male gonad.

THEORY   What a scientist believes is probably so but cannot prove.

THYMUS   A gland, populated largely by lymphocytes, which is located in the chest directly above the heart. Its function is the production of lymphocytes, and it probably has a role in regulating their number. The true function of this organ has not really been clarified as yet. Leukemia in mice often starts there.

TONSILLECTOMY   The surgical removal of the tonsils, along with a small amount of money.

TOXIC   Poisonous—causing injury or death. A substance can be nontoxic in small doses and highly toxic in large ones.

TREATMENT   That which is done in an attempt to cure a disease.

TUMOR   When used as a verb it means swelling, and when used as a noun means a neoplasm (a new growth).

ULCER   A hole in any covering surface; this can be in the skin or digestive tract.

UTERUS   The womb.

VACCINATION   The injection of live or killed microorganisms given in order to prevent a disease.

VERRUCA   A wart. *Verruca vulgaris* is the common wart.

VIVISECTION   A section of, or a cutting operation upon a living animal; as distinguished from surgery which is performed on people.

WATER   The major ingredient of most medicines—and the people that imbibe them.

XERODERMA PIGMENTOSUM   A rare hereditary disease characterized by the presence of brown spots and ulcers of the skin; and the frequent production of skin cancers on exposure to sunlight.

Acknowledgments

Mark Twain, in a letter to Annie Sullivan, the teacher of Helen Keller, said:

> . . . substantially all ideas are second-hand, consciously and unconsciously drawn from a million outside sources, and daily used by the garnerer with a pride and satisfaction born of the superstition that he originated them: whereas there is not a rag of originality about them anywhere except the little discoloration they get from his mental and moral calibre and his temperament, which is revealed in characteristics of phrasing. . . . It takes a thousand men to invent a telegraph, or a steam engine, or a phonograph, or a photograph, or a telephone, or any other important thing—and the last man gets the credit and we forget the others. He added his little mite—that is all he did. . . .
>
> In 1886 I read Dr. Holmes's poems, in the Sandwich Islands. A year and a half later I stole his dedication, without knowing it, and used it to dedicate my "Innocents Abroad" with. Ten years afterward I was talking with Dr. Holmes about it. He was not an ignorant ass—no, not he; . . . and so when I said, "I know now where I stole, but who did you steal it from?" he said, "I don't remember; I only know I stole it from somebody, because I have never originated anything altogether myself, nor met anybody who had.*

I am fully aware that most of the ideas which are expressed here are not original with me. If I could remember where I "stole" them, I would be glad to acknowledge them. In the course of conversations with my colleagues, many of these ideas were probably expressed. With the exception of

* Henney, Nella (Braddy), *Anne Sullivan Macy, The Story Behind Helen Keller* (Garden City, N.Y.: Doubleday, Doran, and Co., 1933), p. 162.

references to publications, I have been unable to acknowledge this assistance. I can only acknowledge those people who have consciously afforded me a large amount of personal help.

My greatest debt is to my parents for the gifts of life and love—and to my father in particular, for teaching me a gentle skepticism.

My training at the Bronx High School of Science was a wonderful experience, due largely to an enthusiastic faculty. I am particularly indebted to Dr. Charles Tanzer, who enjoyed enthusiastic kids, and encouraged them.

At the University of California at Berkeley, my greatest debts are to Dr. Kenneth B. DeOme, who guided my career as a graduate student with kindness, understanding and almost inexhaustible patience and to Dr. Curt Stern for arousing my enthusiasms for genetics (which led to many other things), and for some very valuable lessons in how to be a teacher.

I received two indispensable kinds of help with this book. One kind was the encouragement that was sorely needed after the completion of the first draft. This was provided by Doctors Ernst Eichwald, Herbert B. Fowler, Louis S. Goodman, Bernard I. Grosser, Thomas C. King, Ralph C. Richards, Maxwell M. Wintrobe, Michael B. Shimkin, Richmond T. Prehn, and Meredith N. Runner; Marilyn and Sherman Jensen, and my daughter Anne E. Pilgrim.

The other kind of help is the criticism that made this a better book. The following people reviewed all or parts of the manuscript: Doctors Earl B. Barnawell, Ralph Meader, Charles W. Mays, Robert W. McDivitt, and Robert Zechnich.

I am indebted to them for their help, but would like to make it clear that the opinions expressed in this book are mine.

The writing of this book was supported in part by Research Career Development Award CA19045 from the National Cancer Institute, National Institutes of Health, U.S. Public Health Service.

I am grateful to Miriam Rich and Earleen Porter for their secretarial assistance.

My "Severest Critic and Best Friend" award goes to Theron Raines.

My greatest debt is to my wife—for almost everything else.

References

GENERAL

Ambrose, E. J., and Roe, F. J. C. *The Biology of Cancer*. London and Princeton, N.J.: D. Van Nostrand, 1966. (Fairly technical)

Berenblum, I. *Cancer Research Today*. London: Pergamon Press 1967. Written from the scientist's point of view. Reasonably detailed, but makes fairly easy reading. Particularly valuable to someone with a background in biology.

Cameron, C. S. *The Truth About Cancer*. New York: Collier Books, 1967. A book for the layman written from the point of view of the physician. It has a good deal of information about specific forms of cancer. There is an outstanding section on cancer quackery, and much good advice on things such as breast self-examination.

Foulds, L. *Neoplastic Development*. London: Academic Press, 1969. The historical review in this book is worth reading by the physician or the biologist for an overview of the field of experimental cancer research. It is written for the specialist rather than the layman.

Leighton, J. *The Spread of Cancer*. New York and London: Academic Press, 1967. An excellent book on the spread of cancer (metastasis) written for the professional.

McGrady, Pat. *The Savage Cell*. New York: Basic Books, 1964. Easy reading about cancer research. McGrady is a professional science writer, and it shows. It contains a large amount of information in easily digestible form.

Perez-Tamayo, R. *Mechanisms of Disease: An Introduction to Pathology.* Philadelphia: W. B. Saunders, 1961. A remarkably concise discussion of tumors, intended for the student of pathology and the specialist. It has a very discriminating synthesis of clinical observation and experimental cancer research.

Shimkin, Michael B. *Science and Cancer*, Public Health Service Publication No. 1162, 1969. Very easy reading, highly informative, and concise book—it says an awful lot in 150 pages.

ANYTHING GROWS

(All highly technical)

Leblond, C. P. "Classification of Cell Populations on the Basis of Their Proliferative Behavior," in *Control of Cell Division and the Induction of Cancer*, Monograph 14. Bethesda, Md.: National Cancer Institutes, 1964, pp. 119–149.

Pilgrim, H. I. "The Kinetics of the Organ-specific Metastasis of a Transplantable Reticuloendothelial Tumor." *Cancer Research* 29 (1969): 1200–1205.

The Proliferation and Spread of Neoplastic Cells. Baltimore: Williams and Wilkins, 1968, 794 pages. A collection of papers on the spread and growth of tumors.

WHY TUMORS SEEM WILD

(All technical)

Abercrombie, M., and Ambrose, E. J. "The Surface Properties of Cancer Cells: A Review." *Cancer Research* 22 (1962): 525–548.

Hoffman, J. G., Goltz, H. L., Reinhard, M. C., et al.: "Quantitative Determination of the Growth of a Transplantable Mouse Adenocarcinoma." *Cancer Research* 3 (1943): 237–242.

Huseby, R. A., and Bittner, J. J. "Differences in Adrenal Responsiveness to Postcastrational Alteration as Evidenced by Transplanted Adrenal Tissue." *Cancer Research* 11 (1951): 954–961.

Iversen, O. H. "Kinetics of Cellular Proliferation and Cell Loss in Human Carcinomas: A Discussion of Methods Available for *In vivo* Studies." *European Journal of Cancer* 3 (1967): 389–394.

Laird, A. K. "Dynamics of Tumor Growth: Comparison of Growth Rates and Extrapolation of Growth Curve to One Cell." *British Journal of Cancer* 19 (1965): 278–291.

Pilgrim, H. I. "Studies of Postcastrational Adrenal Cortical Changes in Parabiotic C3H Female Mice." *Cancer Research* 21 (1960): 1555–1560.

Steel, G. G., Adams, K., and Barret, J. C. "Analysis of the Cell Population Kinetics of Transplanted Tumors of Widely Differing Growth Rate." *British Journal of Cancer* 20 (1966): 784–800.

Stohlman, F., Jr., ed. *The Kinetics of Cellular Proliferation.* New York: Grune & Stratton. 1959.

Weiss, P., and Kavanau, J. L. "A Model of Growth and Growth Control in Mathematical Terms. *Journal of General Physiology*, 41 (1957): 1–47.

MAN AS A HOLE

Steinberg, M. "Does Differential Adhesion Govern Self-Assembly Processes in Histogenesis? Equilibrium Configuration and the Emergence of a Heirarchy Among Populations of Embryonic Cells." *Journal of Experimental Zoology* 173 (1970): 395–434. This is a scientist's way of saying what I have described on page 23. The answer to his question "Does differential adhesion govern self-assembly processes in histogenesis?" is *yes!*

This reference, as you might have guessed from the title, is highly technical.

Pilgrim, H. I. "Relationship of the Selective Metastatic Behavior of Tumors of Reticular Tissues to the Migration Patterns of Their Normal Cells of Origin." *Journal of the National Cancer Institute* 49 (1972): 3–6.

NOT ANOTHER BREAKTHROUGH?

The following two references refer to the work of Rous and Huggins that won them the Nobel Prize. They are both fairly technical. •

Rous, F. P. "The Challenge to Man of the Neoplastic Cell" (Nobel Prize Lecture). *Cancer Research* 27 (1967): 1919–1924; also in *Science* 157 (1967): 24–28.

Huggins, C. B. "Endocrine-induced Regression of Cancers" (Nobel Prize Lecture). *Cancer Research* 27 (1967): 1925–1930.

Oberling, Charles. *The Riddle of Cancer*. New Haven, Conn.: Yale University Press, 1944. This book is written by a French scientist and represents the point of view of someone who believes very strongly that cancer is caused by viruses. It is well written, well translated, and makes fairly easy reading. One of the most interesting parts of the book is his discussion of the series of events that led up to Fibiger winning the Nobel Prize, and the events following that indicated that his results were not repeatable. Oberling retains his objectivity throughout the book despite his being an adherent of the virus theory of cancer.

Watson, J. D. *Molecular Biology of the Gene*. New York: W. A. Benjamine, 1965. This is a book for students of molecular biology. Two simpler, more readable books are listed below.

Asimov, I. *The Genetic Code*. New York: New American Library, 1963.

Frankel, E. *DNA—Ladder of Life*. New York: McGraw-Hill, 1964.

STATISTICS

(All technical)

Cancer Facts and Figures. New York: American Cancer Society, published annually.

"Cancer Registration and Survival in California." Berkeley, Calif.: State of California Department of Public Health, California Tumor Registry, 1963.

Connecticut State Department of Health

1964 "Cancer in Connecticut Mortality Data, 1949–1961," 104 pages.

1967 "Cancer in Connecticut Incidence Characteristics, 1935–1962," 97 pages.

1968 "Cancer in Connecticut Survival Experience, 1935–1962," 114 pages.

Cowdry, E. V. *Etiology and Prevention of Cancer in Man*. New York: Appleton-Century-Crofts, 1968. A compilation of a large amount of statistical data on cancer classified by the affected organ. The bibliography should be useful to people interested in cancer epidemiology.

Fraumeni, J. F., and Miller, R. W. "Leukemia Mortality: Downturn Rates in the United States" *Science:* 155 (1967): 1126–1128.

Lilienfeld, A. M., Pedersen, E., and Dowd, J. E. *Cancer Epidemiology: Methods of Study*. Baltimore: Johns Hopkins Press, 1967, 165 pages.

Pearl, R. *Introduction to Medical Biometry and Statistics*. W. B. Saunders, 1923. Philadelphia. This book is the classic in its field. It explains the assumptions that statisticians sometimes take for granted.

CHEMICAL CARCINOGENESIS

Berenblum, I. *Cancer Research Today*. London: Pergamon Press, 1967. A readable and complete discussion of cancer research. An especially fine section of chemical carcinogenesis, which is the author's specialty.

Herbst, L., Ulfelder, H., Poskanzer, C. "Adenocarcinoma of the Vagina; Association of Maternal Stilbestrol Therapy with Tumor Appearance in Young Women." *New England Journal of Medicine* 284 (1971): 878–881. (Technical

Percivall Pott's astute 1775 paper on this subject has been reprinted, thanks to Dr. Michael Potter, in National Cancer Institute Monograph No. 10 (Conference: Biology of Cutaneous Cancer). It makes very interesting reading.

Price, J. M. *Etiology of Bladder Cancer in Benign and Malignant Tumors of the Urinary Bladder.* Edited by E. Maltry. Flushing, N.Y.: Medical Examination Publishing Co., 1971, pp. 189–261. This is an excellent and complete review of the causes of cancer of the bladder. While it is a technical paper, it is fairly easy to read. It contains a very complete bibliography.

Shabad, L. M. "Geograph and Cancer of the Stomach in the U.S.S.R." *Carcinoma of the Alimentary Tract.* Edited by Walter J. Burdette, 1965. (Technical)

Spatz, M., Smith, D. W. E., McDaniel, E. G., Laqueur, G. L. "Role of Intestinal Microorganisms in Determining Cycasin Toxicity." *Proceedings of the Society for Experimental Biology and Medicine* 124 (1967): 691–697. Highly technical; an elegant series of experiments that show how intestinal bacteria can convert a harmless substance into a powerful carcinogen.

Symposium sponsored by the International Union Against Cancer. *Symposium on Carcinogens of Plant Origin. Cancer Research* 28 (1968): Williams & Wilkins. 2233–2396.

TOBACCO IS A DEADLY WEED!

McGrady, Pat. *The Savage Cell.* New York: Basic Books, 1964, 432 pages. His chapter on tobacco and cancer is outstanding.

Smoking and Health—Report of the Advisory Committee to the Surgeon General of the Public Health Service. Washington, D.C.: U.S. Government Printing Office, Health Service Publication No. 1103, 1964, 387 pages. A well-documented book written by a committee.

RADIATION AND CANCER

(All highly technical)

Blum, H. F. *Carcinogenesis By Ultraviolet Light.* Princeton, N.J.: Princeton University Press, 1959.

Brues, A. M. "Critique of the Linear Theory of Carcinogenesis." *Science* 128 (1958): 693–699. A very thorough discussion in which the author concludes that the relationship of radiation to carcinogenesis is probably not linear, and that there is probably a threshold below which no leukemia is induced.

Folley, J. H., Borges, W., and Yamawaki, T. "Incidence of Leukemia in Survivors of the Atomic Bomb in Hiroshima and Nagasaki, Japan." *American Journal of Medicine* 13 (1952): 311–321.

Fraumeni, J. F., Miller, R. W. "Epidemiology of Human Leukemia: Recent Observations." *Journal of National Cancer Institute* 38 (1966): 593–605. A very thorough discussion of leukemia statistics.

Furth, J., and Upton, A. C. "Vertebrate Radiobiology: Histopathology and Carcinogenesis." *Annual Review of Nuclear Science* 3 (1953): 303–337. A fairly complete review of the subject.

Hemplemann, L. H., Pifer, J. W., Burke, G. J., et al.: "Neoplasms in Persons Treated with X-rays in Infancy for Thymic Enlargement. A Report of the Third Follow-up Survey." *Journal of National Cancer Institute* 38 (1967): 317–341. A complete follow-up study of infants that had received thymic irradiation.

Lewis, E. B. "Leukemia, Multiple Myeloma, and Aplastic Anemia in American Radiologists." *Science* 142 (1963): 1492–1494.

Mays, C. W. "Cancer induction in man from internal radioactivity." *Health Physics* 25 (1973): 585–592. A delightfully written short summary of the work which has been done on cancer caused by the ingestion, inhalation or injection of radioactive substances. Mays is one of a group of quiet people who are providing the accurate information which the public needs to become justifiably outraged.

Mays, C. W., and Lloyd, R. D. "Bone Sarcoma Risk for ⁹⁰Sr." 1971, in press.

Moloney, W. C., and Lange, R. D. "Leukemia in Atomic Bomb Survivors II. Observations on Early Phases of Leukemia." *Hematology* 9 (1954): 663–684.

Simpson, C. L., and Hemplemann, L. H. "The Association of Tumors and Roentgen Ray Treatment of the Thorax in Infancy." *Cancer* 10 (1957): 42–56.

EMBRYOS, GENES, AND CANCER

(All technical)

Gurdon, J. B. Transplanted Nuclei and Cell Differentiation. *Scientific American* 219 (1968): 24–35.

Kleinsmith, L. J., and Pierce, G. B. "Multipotentiality of Single Embryonal Carcinoma Cells." *Cancer Research* 24 (1964): 1544–1551.

Stevens, L. C. "Experimental Production of Testicular Teratomas in Mice of Strains 129, A/He, and Their F1 hybrids." *Journal of National Cancer Institute* 44 (1970): 923–929.

Symposium sponsored by the American Cancer Society. "The Developmental Biology of Neoplasia." *Cancer Research* 28 (1967): 1797–1914.

Much of the work on chalones has been done by W. S. Bullough at the University of London and O. H. Iversen at the University of Oslo. A good overall view can be found in the book edited by Teir, H., and Rytomaa, T. *Control of Cellular Growth in Adult Organisms.* London and New York, Academic Press, 1964.

Chalones: Concepts and Current Researches. National Cancer Institute Monograph 38, July 1973. DHEW Publication No. (NIH) 73–425. This volume is a series of up-to-date articles on chalones. It also has a good historical introduction. The papers are highly technical.

YES, VIRGINIA, VIRUSES DO CAUSE CANCER

Clemens, S. (Twain, M.) *Tom Sawyer*, 1875. The classic paper on wart treatment.

(The following are all highly technical)

Giertsen, J. C. "Malignant Testicular Tumors Following Mumps Orchitis." *Acta Pathologica et Microbiologica Scandinavica* 42 (1957): 7–14.

Gross, L. *Oncogenic Viruses*. New York: Pergamon Press, 1961.

Melnick, J. L. 1965 "The Papovavirus Group," in *Viral and Rickettsial Infections of Man*, 4th ed. Edited by Horsfall and Tanner. Philadelphia: J. B. Lippincott Co., 1965, pp. 841–859.

Prehn, R. T. "Tumor-specific Antigens of Putatively Nonviral Tumors." *Cancer Research* 28 (1968): 1326–1330.

Rowe, Wallace P. "1973 Genetic Factors in the Natural History of Murine Leukemia Virus Infection." *Cancer Research* 33: 3061–3068. A fine, highly technical history and discussion of the cancer-virus-gene problem. Rowe and his group perform highly competent virus-cancer research at the National Institute of Allergy and Infectious Diseases; a stone's throw from the political hubbub of the National Cancer Institute.

Symposium sponsored by the American Cancer Society. "Conference on Tumor-specific Antigens." *Cancer Research* 28 (1967): 1275–1459.

EVERYTHING YOU WANT TO KNOW ABOUT SEX AND CANCER

Elliott, R. I. K. "Carcinoma of the Cervix—Basic Research." *The Prevention of Cancer*. Edited by Raven and Roe. London: Appleton-Century-Crofts, 1967, pp. 281–290.

Fergusson, J. D. "Cancer of the Prostate." In *The Prevention of Cancer*. Edited by Raven and Roe. London: Appleton-Century-Crofts, 1967, pp. 257–261.

Griffiths, J. D. "Carcinoma of the Penis." In *The Prevention of Cancer.* Edited by Raven and Roe. London: Appleton-Century-Crofts, 1967, pp. 262–264.

Mirra, A. P., Cole, P., and MacMahon, B. "Breast Cancer in an Area of High Parity: Sao Paulo, Brazil." *Cancer Research* 31 (1971): 77–83.

Rotkin, I. D. "Adolescent Coitus and Cervical Cancer: Associations of Related Events with Increased Risk." *Cancer Research* 27 (1967): 603–617.

Steele, R., Lees, R. E. M., and Kraus, A. S. "Sexual Factors in the Epidemiology of Cancer of the Prostate." *Journal of Chronic Disease* 24 (1971): 29–37.

Wynder, E. L., Cornfield, J., and Schroff, P. D. "A Study of Environmental Factors in Carcinoma of the Cervix." *American Journal of Obstetrics and Gynecology* 68 (1954): 1016–1052.

Wynder, E. L., Bross, I. J., and Hirayam, T. "A Study of the Epidemiology of Cancer of the Breast." *Cancer* 12 (1960): 559–601.

CANCER IMMUNOLOGY

Conceptual Advances in Immunology and Oncology. New York: Harper & Row. Hoeber Medical Division, 1963. This volume contains the papers from a symposium on "Fundamental Cancer Research" held at the M. D. Anderson Hospital and Tumor Institute in Houston, Texas. Among many interesting (and very technical) articles are papers by Hans O. Sjogren (Sweden) and by Karl Habel (U.S.A.) who independently discovered the immunologic differences in polyoma-induced tumors. There is also a paper by R. H. Wilson et al. on treating human cancer with concentrated antibodies.

Jacobs, Barbara B., and Huseby, R. A. "Growth of Tumors in Allogeneic Hosts Following Organ Culture Explanation." *Transplantation* 5 (1967): 410–419.

IS CANCER INHERITED?

Genetics and Cancer. Austin: University of Texas, 1959. Many papers on genetics and cancer.

Macklin, M. T. "Genetic Considerations in Human Breast and Gastric Cancer." In *Genetics and Cancer*. Austin, University of Texas, 1959, pp. 408–425.

Stern, C. *Principles of Human Genetics*. San Francisco: W. H. Freeman and Co., 1960. This is a textbook of human genetics. It is fairly easy to read.

Tokuhata, G. K. "Familial Factors in Lung Cancer and Smoking." In *Genetics and the Epidemiology of Chronic Diseases*. Washington, D.C., U.S. Dept. of Health, Education, and Welfare, 1965, pp. 339–353.

Woolf, C. M. *Investigations on Genetic Aspects of Carcinoma of the Stomach and Breast,* vol. 2, pp. 265–350. Berkeley: University of California Press, 1955.

WHY SOME TUMORS SPREAD

Greene, H. S. N., and Harvey, E. K. "The Relationship Between the Dissemination of Tumor Cells and the Distribution of Metastases." *Cancer Research* 24 (1964): 799–811.

Kinsey, D. L. "An Experimental Study of Preferential Metastasis." *Cancer* 13 (1960): 674–676.

Leighton, J. *The Spread of Cancer. Pathogenesis, Experimental Methods, Interpretations*. New York: Academic Press, 1967.

Pilgrim, H. I. "The Kinetics of the Organ-specific Metastasis of a Transplantable Reticuloendothelial Tumor." *Cancer Research* 29 (1969): 1200–1205.

Wallace, A. C. "Metastasis as an Aspect of Cell Behavior." In *Canadian Cancer Conference, Proceedings of the Canadian Cancer Research Conference in 1960,* vol. 4, pp. 139–165. New York: Academic Press, 1961.

Weiss, P., and Andres, G. "Experiments on the Fate of Embryonic 'Chick' Cells Disseminated by the Vascular Route." *Journal of Experimental Zoology* 121 (1952): 449–487.

Willis, R. A. *The Spread of Tumors in the Human Body*. London: Butterworth & Co., 1952.

Zeidman, I. "Metastasis: A Review of Recent Advances." *Cancer Research* 17 (1957): 157–162.

IS IT CANCER, DOCTOR?

(Both highly technical)

Clark, W. H., Jr., From, L., Bernadino, E. A., et al.: "Histo-genesis and Biologic Behavior of Primary Human Malignant Melanomas of the Skin." *Cancer Research* 29 (1969): 705–726.
Wintrobe, M. M. *Clinical Hematology*, 6th ed. Philadelphia: Lea & Febiger, 1967.

THE DOCTOR SAID, "HE'LL BE DEAD IN A YEAR"—AND HE ISN'T

The following two books document a goodly number of cases of "proved" cancer either that went into long remission, or where the cancers disappeared completely. Many of the cases that have undergone spontaneous remissions and cures have been some of the rarer types of cancer in children, the so-called embryonic tumors.

Boyd, W. *The Spontaneous Regression of Cancer*. Springfield, Ill.: Charles C Thomas, 1966.
Everson, T. C., and Cole, W. H. *Spontaneous Regression of Cancer*. Philadelphia and London: W. B. Saunders, 1966.

WHEN IN DOUBT, CUT IT OUT!

Ackerman, L. V., and del Regato, J. A. *Cancer: Diagnosis, Treatment, and Prognosis*. St. Louis, Mo.: C. V. Mosby Co., 1962.
Berkson, J., Harrington, S. W., Clagett, O. T., et al.: "Mortality and Survival in Surgically Treated Cancer of the Breast: A Statistical Summary of Some Experience of the Mayo Clinic." *Proceedings of the Staff Meetings of the Mayo Clinic*, 1957.
McDivitt, R. W., Stewart, F. W., and Berg, J. W. "Tumors of the Breast." In *Atlas of Tumor Pathology*, 2nd ser., fascicle 2. Washington, D.C.: Armed Forces Institute of Pathology, 1968. This publication contains the type of in-

formation that a pathologist needs to make a diagnosis. There is also a good discussion of the imponderables in treatment, and a table detailing the results of treatment with different types of tumors.

RADICAL SURGERY

Campion, Rosamond. *The Invisible Worm*. New York: Macmillan Co., 1972. This book tells of the personal experience of a woman with breast cancer. She also discusses the experiences of her acquaintances who have had breast cancer. It is a well-written, well thought-out book. She chose to go to George Crile for a lumpectomy. She summarizes her opinion as follows:

"The truth is this: no woman on earth is exactly like any other woman. Even in the thrall of a dread disease, she is unique and must be paid by her doctor the compliment of being allowed partnership, within the proper framework of her illness, in deciding what is the best solution for her own special or even eccentric needs."

Crile, G. *A Biological Consideration of Treatment of Breast Cancer*. Springfield, Ill.: Charles C. Thomas, 1967. Advocates simple surgery and a "common sense" approach to cancer.

Crile, George. *What Women Should Know About the Breast Cancer Controversy*. New York: Macmillan Co., 1973. I read this book while putting the finishing touches on this manuscript. There was no need to change a word in my book because Crile's conclusions and mine are almost the same. Crile writes well, and his understanding of surgery is profound. He does not believe in the efficacy of radical mastectomy, and prefers simple mastectomy or modified radical mastectomy. He does not, as has been implied in a newspaper article that I have read, "advocate" lumpectomy except for the woman who is willing to risk her life to save her breast. He believes that the patient has the right to make his or her own decisions.

He did point out something which I had completely

overlooked: that the amount of money paid to a surgeon by an insurance company is proportional to the amount of work involved rather than the efficacy of the operation. I phoned my local Blue Shield office and found out that a simple mastectomy is twice as lucrative as a lumpectomy or partial mastectomy and that a radical is two and a half times as lucrative as a simple mastectomy.

Fisher, B. "The Surgical Dilemma in the Primary Therapy of Invasive Breast Cancer: A Critical Appraisal." *Current Problems in Surgery*. Chicago: Year Book Medical Publishers, October 1970, 53 pages. A scholarly, complete, and objective review of the literature. This is "must" reading for the surgeon. He concludes that surgeons should continue with their usual method of treatment until the critical trials have been performed; and these trials are long overdue. They have been started in England, and are being started in this country.

LEUKEMIA IN CHILDREN

"Conference on Acute Leukemia and Burkitt's Tumor." *Cancer Research* 27 (1967): 2414–2660. A series of papers on leukemia and Burkitt's tumor.

Holland, J. F. "Progress in the Treatment of Acute Leukemia, 1966." *Perspectives in Leukemia*. New York: Grune & Stratton, 1968, pp. 217–240.

TO TREAT OR NOT TO TREAT

In the journal *Cancer Research*, vol. 29, no. 12 (November 1969) pages 2262–2485, there is a many-authored discussion of the present state of chemotherapy. Good results have been obtained with the following tumors: Choriocarcinoma, Wilms' tumor (a tumor of the kidney that occurs in children), tumors of the testicle, Burkitt's lymphoma (a lymphocytic tumor which also occurs frequently in children), and Hodgkin's disease.

GO TO A CANCER QUACK—IT'S YOUR LIFE

Cameron, C. S. *The Truth About Cancer*. Englewood Cliffs, N.J.: Prentice Hall, 1956; Also New York: Macmillan Co., 1967. His chapter on the cancer quack is a gem.

PREVENTION IS BETTER

Raven, R. W., Roe, F. J. C., eds. *The Prevention of Cancer*. London: Appleton-Century-Crofts, 1967.

THE MIND AND CANCER

Groddeck, Georg. *Das Buch Vom Es*. Vienna: International Psychoanalytischer Verlag, 1923. This book is available in paperback of an excellent translation as *The Book of the It*. New York: New American Library, Mentor Books, 1961. Groddeck has been called the "father of psychosomatic medicine." He was a contemporary of Freud. Although he was a friend and admirer of Freud, he was never a true disciple. He went his own way and made many original observations (see Carl and Sylva Grossman, *The Wild Analyst*. New York: Dell Publishing Co., 1965). Groddeck has no fancy theoretical constructs to obscure his astute observations. He is a humane physician who is also exquisitely perceptive and an excellent writer. The simplicity of this book is not only deceptive, but seductive. In the words of a young friend of mine. "It's a real mind blower."

FEAR

Crile, G. *Cancer and Common Sense*. New York: Viking Press, 1955. This is a wonderful and readable book by a surgeon. It is delightful reading and full of wisdom and understanding. It has raised some hackles by statements such as, "Those responsible for telling the public about cancer have chosen to use the weapon of fear. They have portrayed cancer as an insidious, dreadful, relentless invader. With religious fervor they have fashioned a devil out of cancer. They have bred in a sensitive public a fear that is approaching hysteria. They have created a new disease, cancerphobia, a contagious disease that spreads from mouth to ear. It is possible that today cancerphobia causes more suffering than cancer itself." Page 7.

This book was written at a time surgeons were doing super-radical operations that have now been largely discredited. It is already a classic, and is "must reading" for physicians, patients, and anyone who is interested in disease and the human being.

Kubler-Ross, Elisabeth. *On Death and Dying.* New York: Macmillan Co., 1969. (This is available in paperback) This book is by a psychiatrist who has been working with the terminally ill. It is a very readable book, and should be "must reading" for all physicians and clergymen. It describes how people react to serious illness. One of the underlying themes, which isn't specifically stated, appears to be "Physician, heal thyself." It is a sensitive, wise, and understanding book.

I tried to summarize this book in an attempt to give the reader the essence of what is said in it. I found myself removing so many large quotations, that I would feel that I would have had to pay Dr. Kubler-Ross royalties for taking that much. It is not very useful to try to summarize something that is already said both well and compactly. All that I can recommend, therefore, is that you read the book.

FORGIVING

Anderson, Robert. *After* (a novel). New York: Random House, 1973. Anderson is one of the finest playwrights of our time, and now rates as a novelist. He combines exquisite sensitivity and perception with superb writing craftsmanship. He writes of the ordeal of a man whose wife has died of breast cancer. He relives her dying and his subsequent attempts to adjust to her loss and resume the business of living. His "Christopher Larsen" (his main character) is the brother of every man who has ever lost a wife. The people are alive in this superb novel.

THE CANCER BUCK

The August 1957, vol. 19, no. 2, issue of the *Journal of the National Cancer Institute* is devoted to a history of the National Cancer Institute on the twentieth anniversary of its existence.

Greenberg, Daniel S. 1967. *The Politics of Pure Science*. New York: New American Library. This book is a blistering critique of the politics of "pure science." Greenberg is a science reporter, and an excellent one. The book is perceptive and well written. Greenberg has sniffed out all of the inconsistencies, mistakes, and defects in the scientific establishment. What is missing is love. It would be very easy to point out the idiocies in sex or skiing or any other human endeavor if one had never tried it. This book bears the same relationship to science that a Tennessee Williams play bears to life. It is, nevertheless, a very important book that has much to say to the scientist about the peculiar world in which he lives. Greenberg brings an objectivity to this discussion of science that a scientist might be incapable of. I find myself emotionally opposed to what he says; but what he says is true.

Nisbet, Robert. *The Degradation of the Academic Dogma*. New York: Basic Books, 1971. This book presents a view of what has happened to universities during the years 1945–1970. Nisbet is a sociologist who has a penetrating insight into what has happened during that period of time.

Strickland, Stephen P. *Politics, Science, and Dread Disease*. Cambridge: Harvard University Press, 1972, 317 pages. This book is a "short history of United States medical research policy." It contains the complete story of what has happened in cancer politics since 1927. It is a complete and authoritative work.

CREATIVE FEDERALISM OR BUREAUCRACY

DeBakey. M. E. et al. *A National Program to Conquer Heart Disease, Cancer, and Stroke.* Washington, D.C.: U.S. Government Printing Office, 1964, 644 pages.

"National Cancer Institute Fact Book." *National Cancer Institute,* published annually.

Strickland, S. P. "Integration of Medical Research and Health Policies." *Science* 173 (1971): 1093–1103. A brief, informative, readable article on the history of federal support of medical research.

Wooldridge, D. E. et al. *Biomedical Science and Its Administration: A Study of the National Institutes of Health.* Washington, D.C.: U.S. Government Printing Office, 1965.

Yarborough, R., and Committee. "National Program for the Conquest of Cancer. Report of the National Panel of Consultants on the Conquest of Cancer Authorized by Senate Resolution 376." Washington, D.C.: U.S. Government Printing Office, 1970, 150 pages (#52–532) 91st Congress, 2nd Session.

SCIENTISTS, RESEARCH, AND DISCOVERY

Barber, B. "Resistance by Scientists to Scientific Discovery." *Science* 134 (1961): 596–602.

Chargaff, E. "Preface to a Grammar of Biology." *Science* 172 (1971): 637–642. This is a wonderful, wise, and well-written essay on the "state of the art" of biology. Chargaff is the man who made the discovery of the base ratios in DNA. I thought of reprinting it verbatim, but decided not to because my book might suffer by the comparison.

Dunn, T. B. "The Value of Animal Research, and the Men Who Do this Research." *Cancer Research* 22 (1962): 898–905. A warm and great lady of cancer research talks about people.

Greenberg, Daniel S. *The Politics of Pure Science.* New York: New American Library, 1967.

Stewart, H. L. "The Cancer Investigator." *Cancer Research* 19

(1959): 804–818. A humorous and wonderful essay describing the cancer research scientist's utopia, and the author's personal philosophy—one of the finest bits of literature ever published in a cancer journal.

HOW GOES THE WAR
AGAINST CANCER—AN EDITORIAL

Culliton, Barbara J. "National Cancer Act: Deciding on People, Politics, and Plans." *Science* 176 (1972): 386–390.

—— "National Cancer Plan: The Wheel and the Issues Go Round." *Science* 179 (1973): 1305–1308.

—— "Cancer News: Cancer Society Makes It with Style." *Science* 180 (1973): 722–724.

—— "Biomedical Research 1973: Cancer, Heart Disease, and Everything Else." *Science* 181 (1973): 828–830.

—— "Biomedical Research (II): Will the 'Wars' Ever Get Started?" *Science* 181 (1973): 921–925.

These are a series of articles on cancer politics. The author is an exceptionally well-informed science writer. They are well worth reading. It might help if the directors of the National Cancer Institute and members of Congress read them.

The following three articles are a response to the advocates of a crash program to cure cancer. They were written at the time when Congress was considering creating a new "Cancer Authority." All three are highly critical.

Bazell, Robert. "Behind the Cancer Campaign." *Ramparts*, December 1971.

Eisenberg, Lucy. "The Politics of Cancer." *Harper's Magazine*, November 1971.

Wade, Nicholas. "Special Virus Cancer Program: Travails of a Biological Moon Shot." *Science* 74 (1971): 1306–1311.

INDEX